Ghada Bouslama
Nour Ben Messaoud

Horizontal bone augmentation techniques in implantology

Ghada Bouslama
Nour Ben Messaoud

Horizontal bone augmentation techniques in implantology

news and innovations

ScienciaScripts

Imprint

Any brand names and product names mentioned in this book are subject to trademark, brand or patent protection and are trademarks or registered trademarks of their respective holders. The use of brand names, product names, common names, trade names, product descriptions etc. even without a particular marking in this work is in no way to be construed to mean that such names may be regarded as unrestricted in respect of trademark and brand protection legislation and could thus be used by anyone.

Cover image: www.ingimage.com

This book is a translation from the original published under ISBN 978-620-6-72292-2.

Publisher:
Sciencia Scripts
is a trademark of
Dodo Books Indian Ocean Ltd. and OmniScriptum S.R.L publishing group

120 High Road, East Finchley, London, N2 9ED, United Kingdom
Str. Armeneasca 28/1, office 1, Chisinau MD-2012, Republic of Moldova, Europe
Printed at: see last page
ISBN: 978-620-8-25359-2

Contents

INTRODUCTION

Implant-supported rehabilitation of edentulous teeth, whether partial or complete, is currently considered a highly predictable treatment option, offering reliable long-term results. However, in cases of insufficient bone volume, implant placement may be compromised or even impossible. In such circumstances, a bone augmentation procedure becomes essential to promote implant osteointegration and ensure long-term treatment success.

Insufficient bone depth is a frequent occurrence. These horizontal bone defects can be caused by various pathologies such as periodontitis, infection, trauma or post-extraction bone resorption.

Managing horizontal bone defects can be a challenge for dentists when planning and positioning implants. Several techniques are used to correct horizontal bone defects and ensure successful implant placement. These include the use of guided bone regeneration techniques, autogenous bone apposition grafting and bone expansion to increase bone width by osteotomy.

Each of these techniques has its own advantages and disadvantages, and their selection will depend on the specific needs of the patient and the skills of the practitioner.

The aim of this thesis is to highlight the different techniques for managing horizontal bone defects in dental implantology through the analysis of a series of clinical cases and a recent review of the scientific literature, highlighting the advantages and disadvantages of each approach as well as the scientific evidence supporting their effectiveness. We will also look at the factors that predict the success or failure of the various techniques.

1. ETIOLOGY OF HORIZONTAL BONE DEFECTS

1. ETIOLOGY OF HORIZONTAL BONE DEFECTS

1.1. Alveolar healing and post-extraction resorption

Following dental avulsion, the healing process begins, accompanied by bone resorption of the alveolar bone, which remains an inescapable phenomenon leading to unfavourable pre-implant aesthetic and functional situations.

From the 20th day after extraction, bone neosynthesis is evidenced by the appearance of neoformed bone trabeculae, and osteosynthesis is completed 15 weeks later. This is due to the high level of osteoclastic activity attacking the vestibular and lingual outer surfaces; this alveolysis is more pronounced in the vestibular region than in the lingual/palatal region (Figure 35). Although continuous throughout life, this resorption is greatest in the first few months after extraction, with a reduction in crete width of up to 50% in the first year following the loss of a premolar and molar tooth, or two-thirds of the total changes occurring in the first 3 months post-extraction.(1) (2)

This loss is on average 40% in height and 60% in width of the crete in the 6 months following avulsion. (Agarwa et Al 2012) (2)

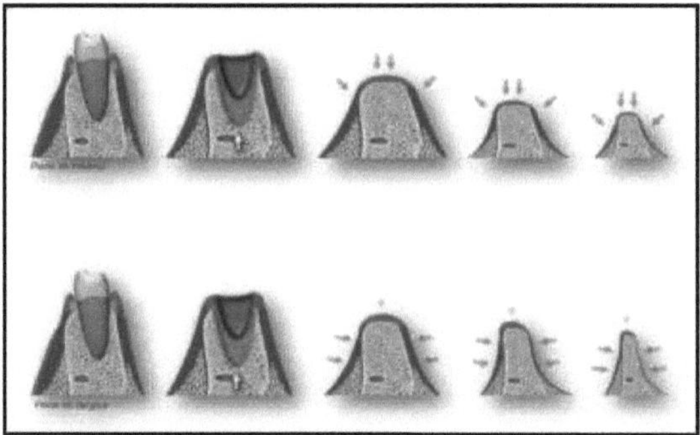

Figure 1. height and width of bone loss after extraction (3)

A study by Sandra Sahur et al (4) in the table below measures average vertical and horizontal bone loss after tooth extraction clinically and radiographically in molar and non-molar sites:

Table I. Representative table of horizontal and vertical bone loss from quantitative analyses (4)

	Non-molar sites			Molar sites		
	Horizontal loss	Vertical loss		Horizontal loss	Vertical loss	
		Vestibular dimension	Lingual dimension		Vestibular dimension	Lingual dimension
Radiology	2.54mm			3.61mm		
		1.65mm	1.44mm		1.46mm	1.20mm
Clinical aspects	2.73mm	1.71mm	1.44mm			

A study of 50 patients by Covani in 2011 showed that alveolysis takes on a very specific pattern; it is produced mainly in the centre of the alveolus, while the proximal mesial and distal areas adjacent to healthy periodontal areas remain almost unchanged at 8 weeks of healing, since they are supported by the periodontal ligament (PDL) of the neighbouring teeth (1) (2).

Post-extraction resorption appears to be influenced by factors such as vestibular cortical thickness and tooth angulation. Cortical thickness is a determining factor, and the thicker the walls, as measured by cone-beam volume tomography, the less bone resorption there is. It has been shown that the vestibular wall of the maxilla in the incisivocanine sector is particularly affected by this phenomenon, as the cortical bone is particularly thin. (1) (2)

In addition, a clinical and radiological study using cone-beam volume tomography showed that post-extraction bone resorption is influenced by periodontal biotype and bone cortical thickness.

In the thin periodontal biotype with cortical bone thickness less than or equal to 1 mm, resorption resulted in a median vertical bone loss of 7.5 mm, equivalent to 62% of the initial facial bone height after 8 weeks of healing (Figure 36). In contrast, in patients with a thick phenotype with a thick cortical bone greater than 1 mm, median vertical bone loss was only 1.1 mm, or 9% (2).

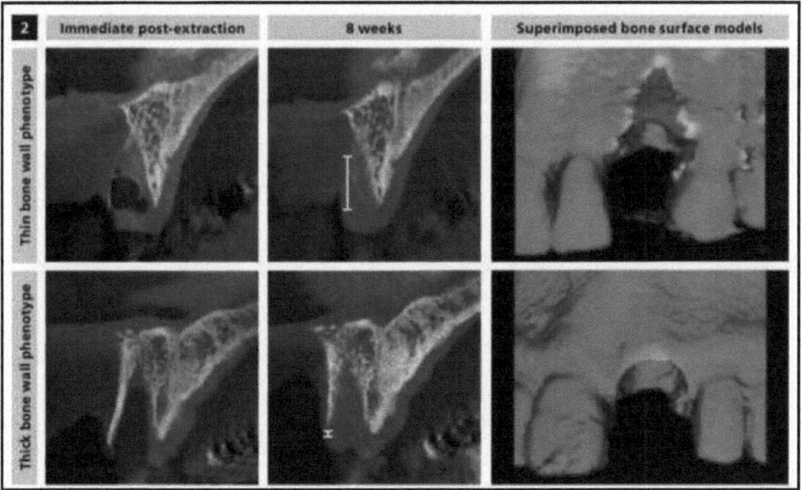

Figure 2. Bone resorption in the thick-walled and thin-walled phenotypes: sagittal sections and 3D images. (2)

1.2. Other causes of bone defects

• **Periodontal disease:** periodontitis is characterised by deterioration of the tissues that support the teeth, mainly including the alveolar bone. Let's assume that diabetes and smoking can be indirect causes of bone defects, since diabetic patients and smokers are frequently prone to periodontal disease.

- **Metabolic bone diseases that disrupt bone metabolism:** hyperparathyroidism, vitamin D-resistant rickets, bone cancer, etc.
Paget's disease, post-menopausal or cortico-induced osteoporosis. (5)
- **Cysts and tumours:** Bone loss is either related to the initial volume and development of the tumour or cyst, or to the surgical procedure, which may result in a post-surgical bone defect.
- **Mutilating surgical procedures:** traumatic extractions, avulsions of impacted teeth, apical resection surgery.
- **Alveolar-dental trauma:** When such trauma occurs, it can lead to significant bone defects in the alveolus, manifested by a loss of bone volume, deformation of the alveolus or bone resorption.
- **Pneumatisation of the maxillary sinus:** is of physiological origin, observed after extraction of the posterior maxillary teeth, and can be explained by the thin cortical bone of the roots of the teeth protruding into the sinus. This cortical bone may be displaced or fractured following dental avulsion, allowing the maxillary sinus to expand. This, together with post-extraction resorption, results in marked bone loss in the posterior bony region (6).
- **Bone defects of congenital origin:** cleft alveoli, micrognatia, oligodontia and agenesis: bone development is linked to the presence of teeth, and in the absence of teeth, there is a bone defect opposite the teeth.

2.
CLASSIFICATION OF BONE DEFECTS

2. CLASSIFICATION OF BONE DEFECTS

Seibert (1983) considered 3 categories in order to classify the different aspects of alveolar bone insufficiency according to their horizontal and vertical components (figure 37):

- **Class I:** Bone defect in the vestibulo-lingual/palatal region with normal bone height. (Horizontal bone loss)
- **Class II:** Corono-apical bone defect with normal bone thickness. (Vertical bone loss)
- **Class III:** Combined bone defect, in the 2 vestibulo-lingual and corono-apical directions. (7)

It should be noted that the prognosis appears to be more favourable in cases of horizontal bone loss (compared to a vertical or combined defect), and less favourable if several teeth are missing or if there is significant loss of attachment to adjacent teeth.

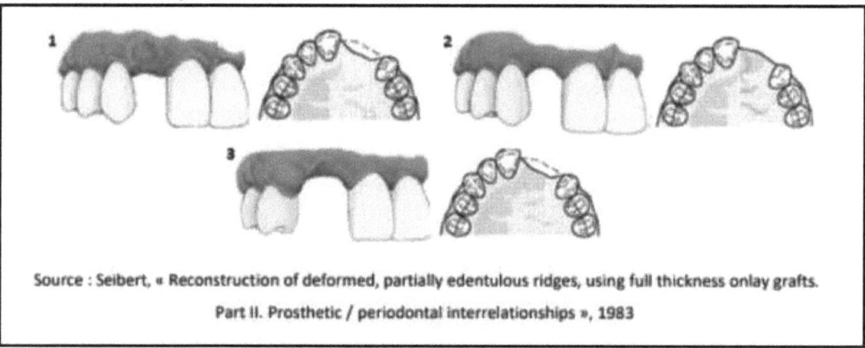

Figure 3: Classification of bone defects according to Seibert 1983 (7)

This classification gives no idea of the quantitative character of the loss, which seems to be an important guide in establishing the treatment plan for the bone defect. Allen et al (1985) therefore suggested a classification based on the degree of severity of the alveolar defect:

- Bone loss < 3mm: **slight**
- Bone loss between 3mm and 6mm: **moderate**
- Bone loss > 6mm: **severe (7)**

It should be noted that there are other classifications of bone deficiencies:

Table II. Summary table of the different classifications of alveolar bone defects (8)

Author and date	Criteria	Advantage	Inconvenient	Classification
Seibert (1983)	Direction of bone loss.		No quantitative assessment of bone loss.	Class I: vestibulo-lingual bone loss + normal crete height. Class II: vertical bone loss + hollow of normal width. Class III: vertical and horizontal bone loss.
Allen (1985)	Degree of bone loss.	More precise.		Bone loss < 3mm: slight 3mm < Bone loss < 6mm: moderate Bone loss > 6mm: severe
Lekholm and Zarb (1985)	Degree of bone loss.	Classification of bone quality.	No appreciation in the vestibulo-lingual direction.	Class A: normal alveolar crete. Class B: slight resorption of the crete. Class C: alveolar bone completely resorbed, basal bone intact. Class D: basal bone resorption.
Cawood and Howell (1988)	The amount of residual bone.	Enjoy the relief of the crete.		Class I: serrated arch. Class II: bone height after avulsion. Class III: rounded ridge of normal height and thickness. Class IV: very thin ridge, normal height. Class V: flat crete, very resorbed. Class VI: negative crete with resorption of basal bone
Jensen (1999)	Residual bone height.		No appreciation in the vestibulo-lingual direction.	Class A: residual bone>10mm, a 10mm implant is completely covered by bone. Class B: 7mm<residual bone<9mm, 70-90% of a 10mm implant is covered by bone. Class C: 4mm<residual bone<6mm, 40-60% of a 10mm implant is covered by bone. Class D: 1mm<residual bone<3mm, 10-30% of a 10mm implant is covered with bone.
Gardella and Renouard (1999)	Evaluation of components : - mesio-distal-vestibulolinguale/pal			Class I : - limited to 1 or 2 teeth -3 or 4 residual bone walls (vestibulo-lingual) - sometimes significant vertical bone loss (A, B, C, D) Class II : (knife edge) - tooth gap limited to 3 or 4 teeth -1 or 2 residual bone walls in vestibulo-lingual direction - type B or C vertical bone loss Class III: slight loss of substance - tooth gap

	atine-vertical dimension.			limited to one or more teeth -3 or 4 residual bone walls in vestibulo-lingual direction - reduced vertical bone loss (A, B)
Wanget Schammari (2005)	The meaning and degree of loss bone.			Horizontal, vertical and combined defects, then each class is defined as small (P<3mm), medium (M, between 4 and 6mm) and large (G>7mm).

3.

PRE-IMPLANT CLINICAL EXAMINATION

3. PRE-IMPLANT CLINICAL EXAMINATION

The aim of implant placement is always to provide both aesthetic and functional prosthetic rehabilitation. It is therefore essential not to design the prosthesis according to the axis of the implant, which is itself determined by the available bone volume. Instead, the implant should be positioned according to the future prosthesis.

When the available bone volume does not allow positioning consistent with the previously studied prosthetic plan, this is referred to as transverse bone volume insufficiency. In cases where the anatomical and prosthetic aspects differ little, it is possible to align them using angled abutments. However, if there are significant discrepancies, surgical techniques will be required to increase the bone volume.

It is therefore essential to diagnose and demonstrate the transverse insufficiency of bone volume in order to ensure the success of the subsequent prosthetic project.

3.1. Anamnese

It is essential that the patient's medical and surgical history be taken first, in order to anticipate the presence of bone defects resulting from diseases that cause resorption.

In addition, certain diseases or habits may contraindicate the use of pre-implant bone grafts, such as smoking, multi-tarred patients with a high risk of infection, non-motivated patients, etc... As a result, other prosthetic solutions should be considered.

It is important to know the cause of tooth loss, as it can be closely linked to bone loss.

For example, the advanced stages of periodontitis (stages 3 and 4) lead to the loss of one or more teeth accompanied by significant bone resorption reaching 50% or more of the alveolar bone (9). Not forgetting the close relationship between periodontal disease, diabetes (10) and smoking (11), the latter of which not only complicates periodontitis and therefore causes very significant bone loss, but also has a negative influence on the quality of post-implant healing, thereby increasing the risk of peri-implantitis.

In order to limit failure, the practitioner must impose recommendations such as: reducing the number of cigarettes as much as possible in patients who smoke (5 cigarettes/day), contacting the doctor treating diabetic patients in order to balance the diabetes.

3.2. Endobuccal examination

It is possible to deduce by inspection or palpation that there is a horizontal bone defect, manifested by a thinning of the alveolar wall with a vestibular depression, clearly perceptible, especially on palpation, if there are still teeth in the immediate vicinity of the deficient area. At an advanced stage, the appearance is that of a "knife-edge" ridge. The greater the number of missing teeth, the more pronounced the horizontal defect.

In some cases, the thick covering mucosa can mask the thin bone and therefore distort the diagnosis of a horizontal bone defect, which is why a radiological examination must be carried out to verify the presence of this defect.

3.3. Radiological examination using cone beam computed tomography (CBCT)

At present, this radiological technique is the gold standard in pre-implant assessment, enabling bone deficiencies to be highlighted, areas for autogenous bone harvesting to be determined, and the anatomical elements to be preserved, such as the maxillary sinus, nasopalatine canal, mandibular canal and chin foramen, to be precisely defined. This is thanks to the oblique coronal sections that it provides, enabling the arches to be viewed in all 3 spatial directions (12).

At present, this technique is used to re-evaluate trabecular bone density, which plays an important role in the choice of horizontal bone augmentation technique. A new classification of bone quality at the site of the future implant was proposed in 2023 based on the cone beam which combines 2 sub-classifications of cortical bone and cancellous bone as follows: cortical bone is classified according to the thickness of the vestibular cortex, cancellous bone is classified according to radiological density. This gave us 9 classifications (figure 35)

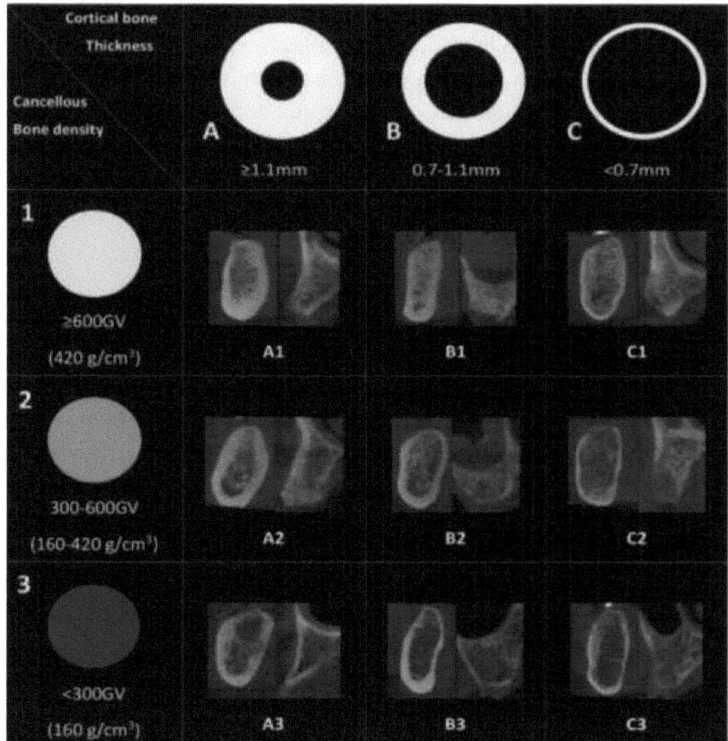

Figure 4. The new bone classification; three different thicknesses (A, B and C) of cortical bone and three different densities (1, 2 and 3) of cancellous bone (13).

In addition, the CBCT examination with DICOM format files offers the practitioner the possibility of reconstructing his or her own images, navigating in the acquired volume and simulating implant placement on 3D reconstructions using digital planning software, while respecting the safety distances required for correct implant positioning.

These safety distances represent one of the bases of the pre-implant analysis which can confirm the existence of a bone defect. They correspond to the bone volumes which must be preserved around the implant in the 3 directions of space, without forgetting to take into account the diameter of the implant chosen. (14)(15)

In the vestibulo-lingual direction, it is imperative to maintain a distance of 1mm vestibularly and lingually in order to guarantee acceptable vascularisation to allow osteointegration of the implant (figure 38). In the maxillary anterior region, 2mm should be left in this direction, as this region is more prone to centripetal resorption (14).

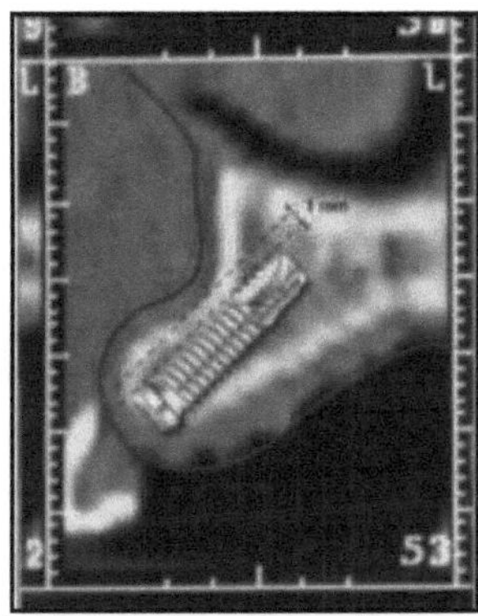

**Figure 5. Vertical and vestibulo-lingual positioning
along the prothetic axis with 1 mm of vestibular bone (14)**

Digital planning therefore makes it possible to estimate the available bone volume according to the position and diameters of the implants and, as a result, several cases may be encountered: (16)(17)

• The prosthetic solution is in line with the underlying bone volume: this is the ideal situation for implant placement.

• The prosthetic plan is not perfectly in line with the available bone volume: in this case, solutions such as idealising the position of the implant, using prosthetic tricks or indicating pre-implant surgery to correct the bone defect should be used.

• The prosthetic plan and the bone volume are in total disagreement: in other words, there is a real bone defect. Bone reconstruction techniques must therefore be considered beforehand, in order to increase bone volume to allow implants to be placed, or to use alternative therapies to implantology, such as conventional dental prostheses (16).

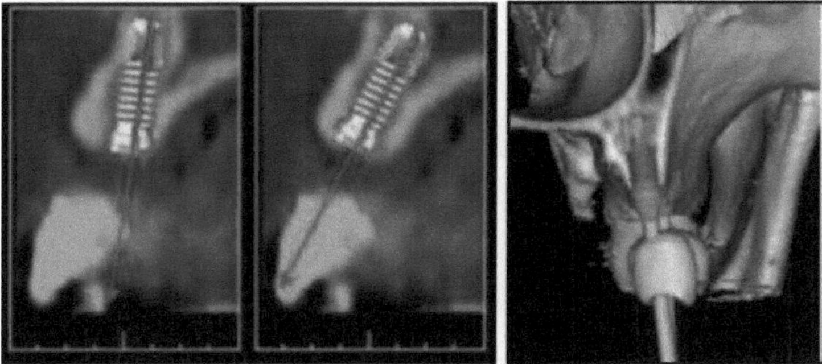

Figure 6. Numerical simulation of implant positioning as a function of the prosthetic project (16)

4.
AUGMENTATION TECHNIQUES HORIZONTAL BONE

4. HORIZONTAL BONE AUGMENTATION TECHNIQUES
4.1. Guided bone regeneration (GBR)

This is the most documented and widely used surgical technique in implantology, and was first described in the 90s by Hurley et al, with protocols evolving over the next 30 years (Figure 38). (18)

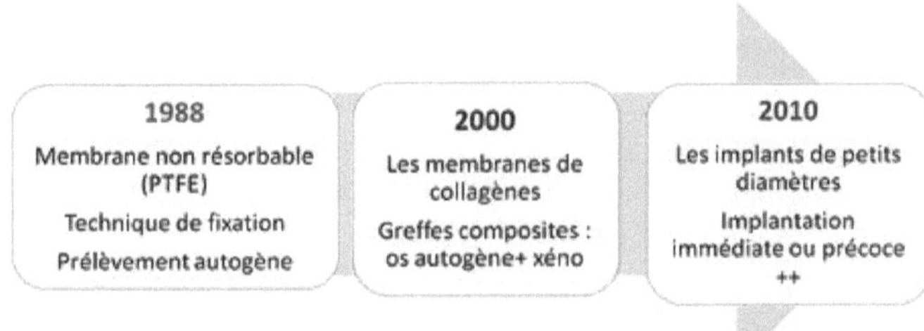

Figure 7. Development of GBR since the late 1980s (18)

ROG increases bone volume via barrier membranes that serve to provide a space conducive to osteogenesis. These membranes are combined with bone filling materials that play a role in optimising bone neoformation and maintaining the scar space (Figure39) (18) (19).

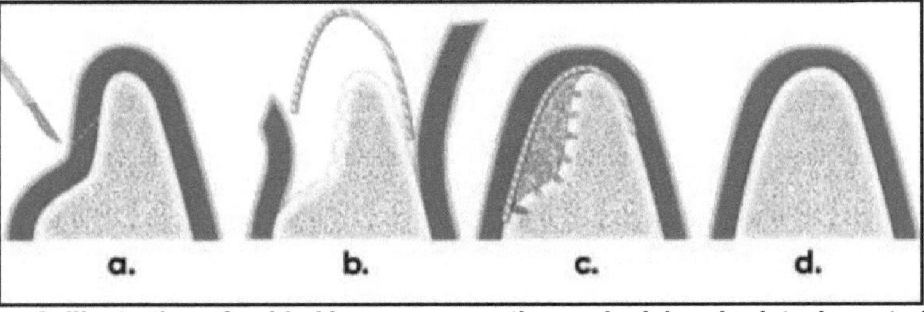

Figure 8: Illustration of guided bone regeneration: a: incision; b: detachment of the flap and insertion of the membrane; c: filling of the space with a bone substitute + insertion and fixation of the membrane using pins + closure of the wound; d: bone neoformation and correction of the bone defect (20).

4.1.1. Biological principle

The biological principle of ROG derives from the same principle of guided tissue regeneration (GTR), which is based on the notion of cell exclusion. In fact, it is accepted that the cells that first populate the area of a wound determine the type of tissue that will eventually occupy the original space, according to the "first come, first served" principle. In this way, the principles of RTG have been applied to the regeneration of bone tissue, and a large series of animal experiments and clinical studies have shown that once the bone defect has been isolated by a physical barrier, provided it is not exposed to the oral environment, optimal conditions then exist for the growth of blood vessels in the resident bone, allowing stem cells and osteoprogenitor cells to differentiate into osteoblasts, which produce the bone matrix and there will therefore be bone neoformation at this level. (18) (19)

The success of guided bone regeneration is based on compliance with the biological principles known as PASS (figure 41). (21) (22)

• **Maintaining a scar space** with sufficient vascular supply to guarantee bone neoformation.

• **The stability of the initial blood clot**, which will be at the origin of the bone regeneration process.

• **The exclusion of non-osteogenic cells** from the gingival connective tissue and epithelium, which would compete with the desired bone neoformation, by setting up a physical barrier.

• **Tension-free gingival sutures** to ensure wound stability and mucosal healing by 1er intention.

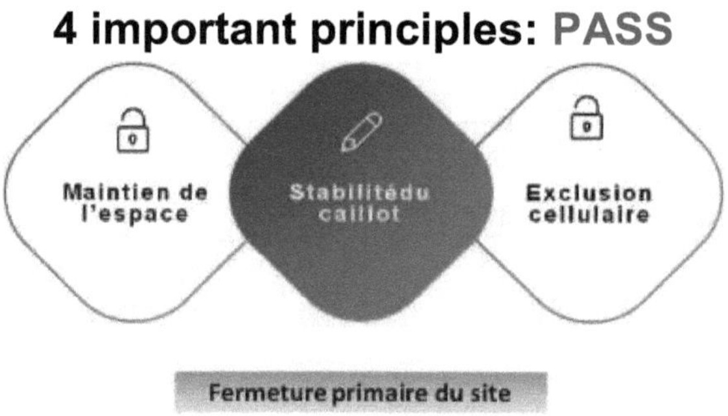

4 important principles: PASS

Maintien de l'espace

Stabilité du caillot

Exclusion cellulaire

Fermeture primaire du site

Figure 9. The 4 biological principles of ROG (21)

4.1.2.   The ROG elements

4.1.2.1.   Membranes

This membrane has 3 main roles: (18) (19)

• **Mechanical role**: To create a suitable space for bone to form. It must therefore be sufficiently rigid to maintain this space.

• **Physical role**: acts as a filter, inhibiting the passage of epithelial and connective cells, while allowing vascularisation and healing mediators to pass through.

• **Role of a** blood clot **stabiliser** and filling material.

There is a wide range of membranes available for guided bone regeneration procedures, these materials meet basic requirements and characteristics such as:

• Biocompatibility.

• Cell exclusion.

- The ability to create a space and maintain it.
- Tissue integration.
- Degradability.
- Ease of clinical handling.
- Susceptibility to complications(18)(19)

These barrier membranes are classified into 2 types: non-absorbable membranes and absorbable membranes (table). Resorbable membranes are further classified, according to their origin, into natural membranes and synthetic membranes.

Table III. Different types of membrane used in ROG procedures(19)

Non-resorbable membranes	Resorbable membranes	
	Natural	Synthetic
e-PTFE (expanded polytetrafluoroethylene) d-PTFE (dense polytetrafluoroethylene) Titanium membrane	Native collagen Collagen reticule	Polyglactine Polyurethane Polylactic acid Polyglycolic acid Copolymers of polylactic acid and polyglycolic acid Polyethylene gylcol

▶ **Non-resorbable membranes**

The most commonly used non-absorbable membranes are e-PTFE (expanded polytetrafluoroethylene) membranes, which were developed in 1960.

The hydrophobic and chemically inert nature of PTFE also makes this biomaterial non-absorbable. In fact, it is resistant to enzymatic degradation by host tissues and microbes, and does not induce inflammatory immunological reactions. The major advantage lies in its excellent barrier function in contact with the bone defect (18)(19).

The membrane is also characterised by its porous structure, which is obtained by exposing the PTFE to high tensile stress, causing it to expand and form a porous microstructure. In addition, the e-PTFE membrane is composed of 2 parts which differ in their density: the denser part is the internal (central) part, located opposite the bone defect, with a pore size of less than 8 pm to allow fluid exchange while preventing the infiltration of undesirable epithelial and connective cells. In contrast, the microstructure of the outer part, which will be in contact with the bone at the edge of the defect, is less dense, containing pores 20 to 25 pm wide and a surface structure that favours the adhesion of blood clots and the attachment of soft connective tissue to the membrane, ultimately leading to tissue integration. (18)(19)

d-PTFE: High Density PTFE differs from e-PTFE in that it contains pores on a submicron scale (0.2 pm), so bacterial infiltration and adhesion will be eliminated due to its high density and small pore size. Furthermore, in the presence of d-PTFE, soft tissue closure becomes unnecessary, as it provides tissue healing with a barrier membrane safely exposed to the oral cavity, limiting the risk of infection after membrane exposure (18)(19).

Indeed, an increased rate of soft tissue complications following premature exposure of the membrane has been reported as a disadvantage of using e-PTFE membranes, not to mention their difficult handling due to their hydrophobic nature, and problems with membrane collapse. Once exposed to the oral cavity, the porous surface of e-PTFE membranes is rapidly colonised by oral microbes.

This often leads to infection of adjacent tissues and the need for early removal of the membrane, which impairs bone regeneration (19).

In addition, PTFE membranes are not rigid enough to maintain the scar space. To overcome this problem of collapse, the PTFE membrane can be mechanically stabilised with titanium, known as titanium-reinforced PTFE. Alternatively, metal mesh membranes made of titanium or an alloy of titanium and a cobalt-chromium alloy can be used (18)(19).

Nowadays, with the advent of digitalisation and three-dimensional printing technology, other techniques are now available to better guarantee space maintenance, customised, three-dimensional (3D) and pre-shaped barrier membranes with favourable mechanical properties are being developed to guarantee ideal bone regeneration. Advances in modern 3D computer-aided planning and the application of computer-aided design or computer-aided manufacturing (Oberoi et al., 2018) have facilitated the fabrication of customised titanium (Ikawa et al., 2016), polyetherethercetone (PEEK) (El Morsy et al., 2020), unsintered hydroxyapatite/poly-L-lactide (uHA/PLLA) (Matsuo et al., 2010) and zirconia to closely fit the anatomical shapes of bone defect areas to better maintain space and achieve accurate volume reconstruction (Vaquette et al., 2021).

However, the major disadvantage of the non-absorbable membrane is the need for a second operation to remove the membrane, which is associated with patient morbidity and the risk of tissue damage during the operation.

Resorbable membranes have been developed to overcome these drawbacks and simplify surgical protocols.

▶ Resorbable membranes (18)(19)

Bioresorbable or biodegradable membranes degrade in the body and disappear over time. They therefore have the advantage of eliminating the need for additional surgery to remove the membrane and expose the regenerated bone.

There are two main categories of bioresorbable membranes: synthetic polymers and polymers derived from various animal sources. Each category has distinct physicochemical properties and biological effects. What interests us most is the degradation process of these membranes, which has an important influence on the outcome, because if degradation occurs too quickly, the membrane would no longer be able to perform its barrier function, and the degradation products may contribute to unfavourable tissue reactions, including foreign body reactions, which may impëcher tissue integration, wound healing and bone formation, or even тёте lead to resorption of already existing bone. In some cases, these reactions can even interfere with the patient's health.

In addition, the lack of rigidity of resorbable membranes means that in some cases it is necessary to add a device to maintain the scar space.

Most bioresorbable membranes used in clinical practice are made from processed collagen or aliphatic polyesters.

❖ Synthetic membranes (18)(19)

The use of synthetic resorbable membranes made from aliphatic polyesters such as polylactic acid (PLA), polyglycolic acid (PLGA), trimethylcarbonate and their copolymers has proved effective for guided bone regeneration procedures in experimental studies, as well as in clinical trials.

However, these synthetic biomaterials have both advantages and dlsadvantages. These advantages include the ability of PGA, PLA and their copolymers to biodegrade completely into carbon dioxide and water via the Krebs cycle. What's more, these biomaterials can be manufactured in almost unlimited quantities.

In a recent multicentre trial involving 40 patients with peri-implant dehiscence, guided bone regeneration was performed using either PLGA or titanium-reinforced e-PTFE membranes. After 6 months at re-entry surgery, mean vertical defect filling was 81% in the PLGA group and 96% in the e-PTFE group. The titanium-reinforced e-PTFE membranes were able to maintain the horizontal thickness of the regenerated region more effectively and developed fewer soft tissue complications than the PLGA membranes.

In addition, PLGA membranes applied to large peri-implant defects appear susceptible to fracture, indicating that the mechanical stability of the membrane is insufficient for this type of application.

A new approach, aimed at simplifying clinical handling, has been adopted with an in situ polymerising synthetic membrane made from polyethylene glycol (figure 42). In situ, polyethylene glycol is degraded by hydrolysis without acid by-products, which have been shown to be responsible for foreign body reactions in surrounding tissues. Preclinical studies have indicated that this material is highly biocompatible and occlusive for cells, and that it allows the formation of similar quantities of new bone compared with other types of material, such as e-PTFE and polylactic acid.

Nevertheless, the use of these membranes as barriers has been associated with inflammatory reactions to foreign bodies due to the degradation products. In some cases, debridement and removal of the biomaterial by means of additional surgery becomes necessary. In addition, some studies have found a reduction in defect filling when polylactic acid and polyglycolic acid membranes are applied compared with collagen membranes.

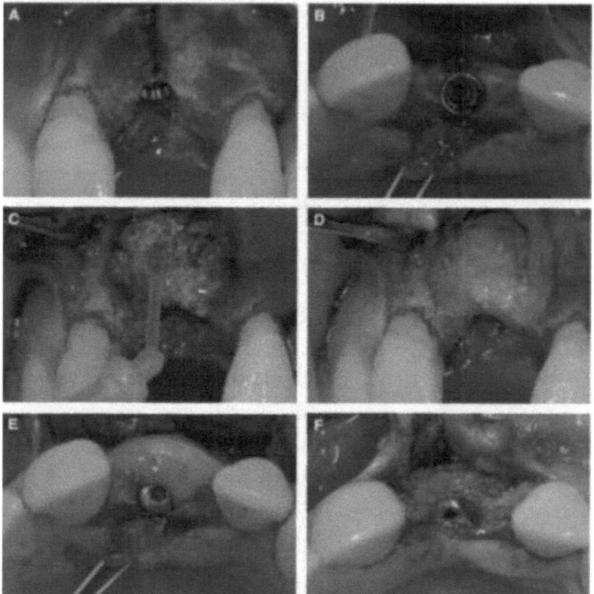

Figure 10 (A, B) Dehiscence-type bone defect at implant position 21 (C) The defect is treated by guided bone regeneration using bovine particulate bone mineral and a polyethylene glycol-based synthetic hydrogel (D, E) Polyethylene glycol membrane polymerised in situ. (F) Re-entry surgery 6 months after implant placement(19)

As a result, collagen membranes are currently recommended over synthetic membranes for guided bone regeneration (GBR) procedures.

*** Natural membranes (18)(19)**

Most natural resorbable membranes are made from collagen derived from animal tissue, although human sources are also available. These collagen membranes come from a variety of tissue sources, including bovine tendon, bovine dermis, calf skin, porcine dermis and human cadaver skin.

Native collagen membranes have good tissue integration, allowing rapid vascularisation and biodegradation without foreign body reaction. In addition, native collagen membranes have shown good results and low complication rates in animal and human studies.

Currently, native collagen membranes are the standard treatment for the majority of indications for guided bone regeneration. Another advantage of using native collagen membranes for guided bone regeneration is spontaneous healing in the presence of mucosal dehiscence. Unlike non-absorbable membranes, in cases of exposure, epithelialisation of exposed collagen results in spontaneous secondary wound closure.

The main disadvantages of native collagen membranes may be due to their unfavourable mechanical properties, such as low resistance to collapse, and their rapid degradation, which leads to an early loss of barrier function. The rapid biodegradation of native collagen by enzymatic activity in host tissues and microbes has been demonstrated in animal models. However, it is important to stress that the degradation time of native collagen can vary considerably depending on its source and original structure.

To extend the barrier function, and therefore the degradation time of the membranes, several physical, chemical and enzymatic cross-linking processes have been developed, such as the use of ultraviolet light, formaldehyde, glutaraldehyde, diphenylphosphoryl azide and hexamethylene diisocyanate, giving rise to cross-linked collagen membranes.

Although increasing the degree of cross-linking prolongs the biodegradation time of the membranes, experimental studies on rats have shown that cross-linking has a negative effect on tissue integration and thus provokes inflammatory reactions to the foreign body. For example, biodegradation of cross-linked collagen membranes by glutaraldehyde leaves cytotoxic residues responsible for inflammatory reactions. In addition, histological studies have shown that inflammatory cells are involved in the resorption process of cross-linked collagen membranes, this may explain the increased frequency of mucosal dehiscence with impaired soft tissue healing and wound infections that have occurred in clinical trials.

Table IV. Comparative table between native and reticulated collagen. (18)

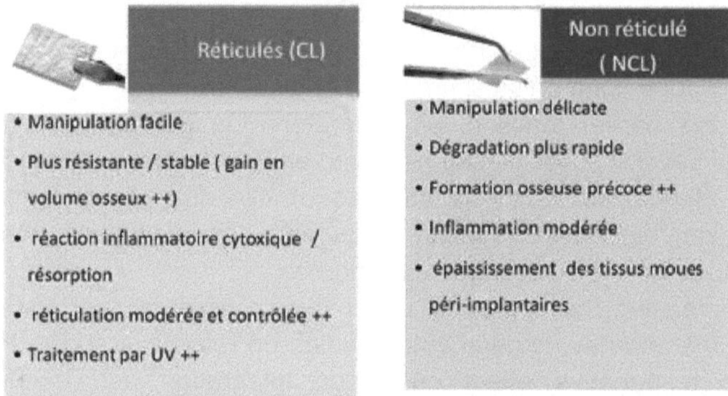

On the other hand, other preclinical and clinical studies have shown promising results for cross-linked collagen membranes, with adequate tissue integration and successful bone regeneration, similar to or even superior to those obtained with native collagen membranes such as ultraviolet light cross-linked membranes. Similarly, several studies have shown that premature exposure of a cross-linked collagen membrane was followed by complete spontaneous secondary epithelialisation without alteration of bone regeneration. These contradictory results indicate differences in biological behaviour between the different types of cross-linked membranes, depending essentially on the cross-linking protocol used(19).

In conclusion, non-reticulated collagen membranes, i.e. native collagen membranes, are currently the membranes of choice for

most guided bone regeneration procedures. Likewise for reticulated collagen membranes, which offer greater stability and scar space maintenance.

4.1.2.2. Bone filling materials (18) (19)

Since most bioresorbable membranes and, to a lesser extent, ePTFE membranes, generally have insufficient rigidity to maintain the defect space, they are often used in combination with autogenous bone grafts, bone substitutes or composite grafts, as is the case when the bone defect exceeds 1mm. In addition to their ability to maintain the defect space, bone fillers fulfil other important functions:

• Providing mechanical support to prevent membrane collapse
• Stabilising the blood clot
• Act as a bone-conducting structure, providing an increased solid base to promote bone growth.
• Possibly have bone-inducing properties due to the presence of proteins

(BMP) which promote and facilitate the multiplication and differentiation of non-specialised stem cells into osteoblasts.

• Have osteogenic properties: by the bone cells of autogenous bone (bone revëtement cells, osteoblasts, stem cells not specialised in osteoblasts and/or osteocytes) which are capable of directly or indirectly promoting bone formation at the graft site.

In addition, filling materials and bone substitutes must meet other conditions such as biocompatibility, the need to provide adequate mechanical support and biodegradability.

Clinical indications for the use of bone filling materials range from the correction of minor peri-implant bone defects to the regeneration of major bone loss. Given this diversity of applications, it is likely that a single material will not be able to meet all requirements. Therefore, it will frequently be necessary to combine two or more materials to obtain a predictable and reproducible result.

Bone filling materials can be derived from the patient himself: autogenous bone grafts, or from an external source classified as allogenic bone substitutes from another individual of the same species, xenogenic from another species and alloplastic: synthetics (Figure 43). These materials come in various forms, such as blocks, granules, mouldable, injectable or in situ hardening materials.

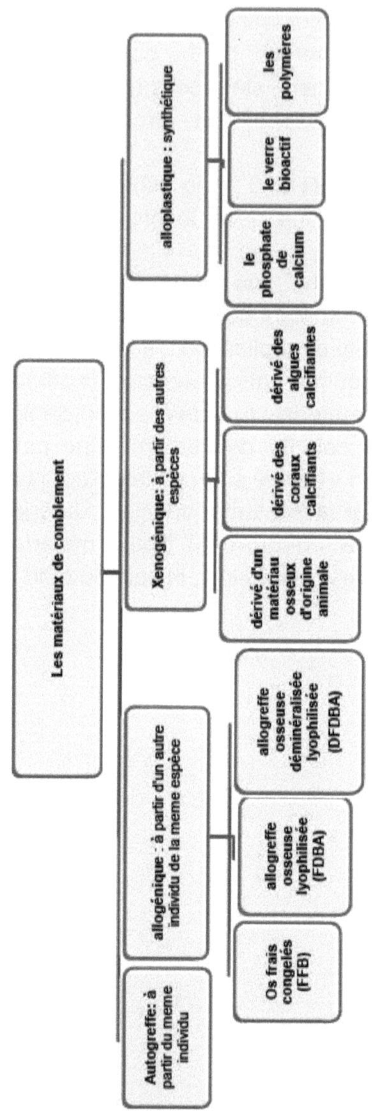

Figure 11. Classification of ROG filling materials (18)

► Autografts (18)(19)

The addition of autogenous bone is preferred because of its osteoinductive, osteogenic and osteoconductive properties. However, autogenous bone harvesting may require additional surgery, resulting in increased operating time, pain and recovery time. In addition, this method is associated with an increased risk of donor site complications, such as increased post-operative pain and nerve damage. In addition, the supply of autogenous bone may be limited.

Through the addition of autogenous bone, viable osteogenic bone cells and bone growth factors are delivered to the recipient site. The quantity of cells and the concentration of growth factors vary considerably from person to person and depend largely on the patient's age, the presence of systemic diseases and the location of the donor site. Growth factors, including BMPs, TGF-в, IGF, PDGF and FGF, are mainly present in the bone matrix. They are released passively or during resorption of autogenous grafts. Cancellous bone blocks release growth factors more rapidly than compact bone blocks. Bone-forming cells, such as osteoblasts, bone lining cells, preosteoblasts and pluripotent stem cells, are the main cells of interest in ROG procedures. They are present in greater numbers in trabecular bone than in compact bone.

Bone formation potential is higher in young, healthy individuals than in the elderly, mainly due to a reduction in the proliferative capacity of bone-forming cells in the latter.

At present, it is recommended to perform a combined filling as follows: 1/3 autogenous bone and 2/3 bone substitute.

xenogenics to optimise bone regeneration results.

► Allogenic bone substitutes: (18)(19)

Allografts consist of bone from a donor and are used in a member of the same species. These allografts are usually stored in bone banks and can be used as fresh frozen bone (FFB), freeze-dried bone allograft (FDBA) or freeze-dried demineralised bone allograft (DFDBA). FFB is rarely used in ROG procedures due to the high risk of immunological rejection and disease transmission. However, freeze-drying FDBA and DFDBA appears to reduce the immunogenicity of the material, potentially improving clinical outcomes. Allografts are available in the form of blocks or particles, of both cortical and cancellous origin. FDBA and DFDBA have been shown to be biocompatible and contain osteoinductive molecules such as BMPs.

Unlike the limitations of autografts, donor site morbidity is not a problem with allografts, and they are available in abundant quantities. However, resorption seems to occur, as with autografts.

In addition, case series have demonstrated that block allografts, combined with resorbable membranes, can be a reliable therapeutic option for augmentation of atrophic alveolar crests in two-stage implant procedures. In a recent clinical trial involving 40 patients, the use of freeze-dried bone block allografts and collagen membranes for primary augmentation of the atrophic maxilla was evaluated. After 6 months, bone samples were harvested and 83 implants were placed. Histomorphometric analysis showed that the mean percentage of newly formed bone was 33 +/- 18% and that of residual allograft was 26 +/- 17%. The implant survival rate was 98.8% after an average follow-up of 48 +/- 22 months.

► **Xenogenic bone substitutes: (18) (19)**

Xenogenic materials, or xenogenic bone substitutes, are made up of bone minerals from animals, calcifying corals or algae, from which the organic component has been removed to prevent immune reactions and the transmission of disease.

Currently, the use of coralline hydroxyapatite as an onlay graft in ROG procedures is rare due to a high rate of late complications and most xenografts are derived from natural sources of bone in animals, in particular bovine cancellous bone is used due to its similarity to human cancellous bone. Organic material is removed by heat treatment, chemical extraction or a combination of both to reduce the risk of immunological reactions and disease transmission. Despite the potential risk of organic residues in bovine bone substitutes, no cases of disease transmission have been associated with the use of these biomaterials. However, a few cases of transmission of HIV and hepatitis attributed to allogenic sources have been reported.

Bovine xenografts are considered to be the best documented bone substitute used in implant dentistry, and are currently accepted as the gold standard. The biocompatibility and osteoconductivity of bovine deprotein bone mineral have been demonstrated in several preclinical studies and clinical case series, and they can be used as bone substitutes without interfering with the normal bone repair process.

In a clinical study, bovine deprotein bone mineral blocks and collagen membranes were applied to 12 patients to treat horizontal bone defects prior to implant placement (Figure 44). After 9-10 months, in 11 of the 12 patients, the resulting bone volume was sufficient to allow implant placement in the prothetically optimal position. It was therefore concluded that the procedure was effective for horizontal augmentation.

However, it should be noted that production processes have a considerable impact on their biological characteristics. For example, high-temperature treatment has been associated with reduced bone formation and reduced osteoconductivity.

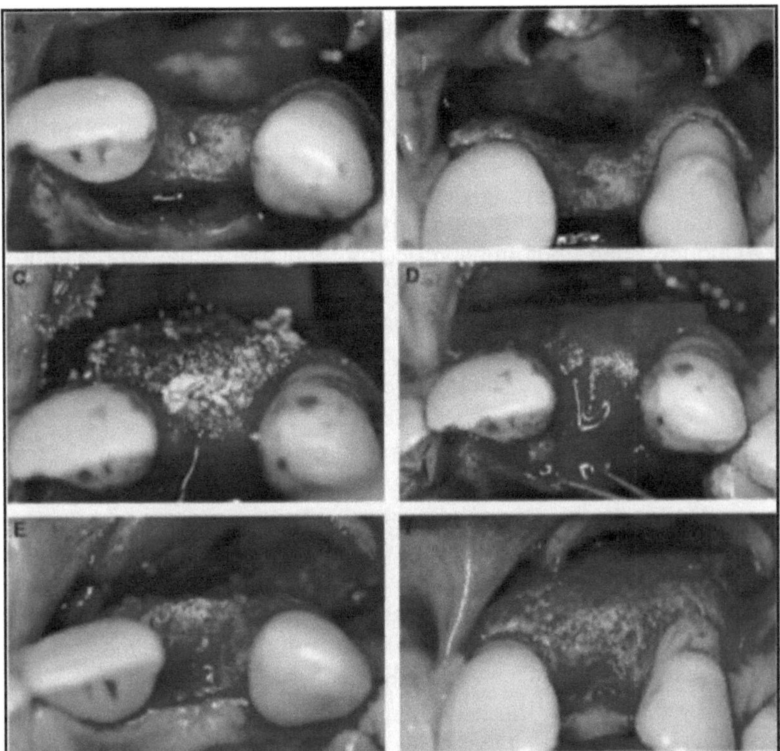

Figure 12: (A,B) Presence of a horizontal bone defect at an implant site 22. (C, D) A block of bovine bone mineral is placed to support a resorbable collagen membrane. (E, F) At re-intervention 9 months later, the volume of the crete was sufficient to allow placement of an implant in the prothetically ideal position (19).

The influence of the granulometry of materials on their resorption time is a crucial element to take into account. It has been shown that particle size must be between 250 and 800 p to guarantee optimum resorption time, thus favouring the neoformation of good quality bone tissue. However, a particle size below 250 p would lead to too rapid resorption, thus compromising the expected supportive role. Similarly, particles larger than 800 p would induce slow resorption, resulting in a delay in the healing process and the formation of poorer quality bone tissue.

► **Alloplastic substitute materials: (18) (19)**

Alloplastic or synthetic bone substitutes offer the advantage of presenting no risk of disease transmission, and are readily available in large quantities.

In addition, these synthetic materials represent a large group of chemically diverse biomaterials, including calcium phosphate (e.g. tricalcium phosphate; hydroxyapatite and calcium phosphate cements), calcium sulphate, bioactive glass and polymers. These materials vary in structure and chemical composition, as well as in mechanical and biological properties.

29

Porous calcium phosphates represent a wide range of bone substitutes available on the market. In addition, they can be a valuable alternative for healthcare professionals and patients who do not wish to use grafts of human or animal origin. Hydroxyapatite is the main mineral component of natural bone and the least soluble of the natural calcium phosphate salts. It is therefore highly resistant to physiological resorption. In contrast, tricalcium phosphate is characterised by rapid resorption and replacement by host tissue. Although bone neoformation occurs regularly in the area intended for regeneration, this neoformation does not fully compensate for the resorption of tricalcium phosphate, resulting in a reduction in the increased volume.

To this end, biphasic compounds of hydroxyapatite and tricalcium phosphate have been developed to combine the advantages of hydroxyapatite and tricalcium phosphate, known as biphasic calcium phosphates (BCP). Preclinical studies using different experimental models have provided histological evidence that particulate or mouldable in situ-hardening hydroxyapatite/tricalcium phosphate has similar osteoconductivity and resorption properties to bovine deprotein bone mineral. A study compared hydroxyapatite/tricalcium phosphate and bovine deprotein bone mineral, in combination with collagen membranes, for guided bone regeneration of extraction alveoli (137). After 8 months, the bucco-buccal dimension of the alveolar crete decreased by 1.1 mm in the hydroxyapatite/tricalcium phosphate group and by 2.1 mm in the bovine deprotein bone mineral group, with a statistically significant difference. Another study showed that hydroxyapatite/tricalcium phosphate gave similar results to bovine deprotein bone mineral for guided bone regeneration of peri-implant dehiscence. In conclusion, on the basis of these results, the combination of hydroxyapatite/ tricalcium phosphate for alveolar crete augmentation is promising for the future.

Table V. Summary table of the different filling materials used in ROG procedures (3)

Features	Autograft	Allografts	Xenografts	Alloplastic grafts
		Bone substitutes		
Content and properties	-Bone matrix Bone-forming cells -Growth factors	-Despecified bone matrix -No Cells -Growth factors (+/-)	-Inorganic mineral matrix! see despecified -No cells -No growth factors	-No cells - No growth factors
	-Need for a second operating site	-Available at -Using bone banks. -Average to good mechanical properties. -Easier handling. /	-Available at - Average mechanical properties /	-Available at - Good mechanical properties /

Osteogenic	+/'	-	-	-
Osteoinductor	+	+/-	-	-
Osteoconductor	+	+	+	+

► Interet d'ajout des facteurs de croissance avec les materiaux de comblements

Clinical studies have shown that the combined use of platelet-rich plasma (PRF) bone grafts and bone particles in regeneration procedures gives promising results. In addition, one study showed that the combination of PRF and bovine deprotein bone blocks in horizontal bone augmentation resulted in an average bone graft stability of 84.4% over a shorter follow-up period of 5 to 8 months.

FRP is rich in growth factors such as PDGF, TGF- pl, IGF and VEGF, which are known to improve angiogenesis, optimise soft tissue healing, stimulate stem cell migration and allow proliferation and osteogenic differentiation (23).

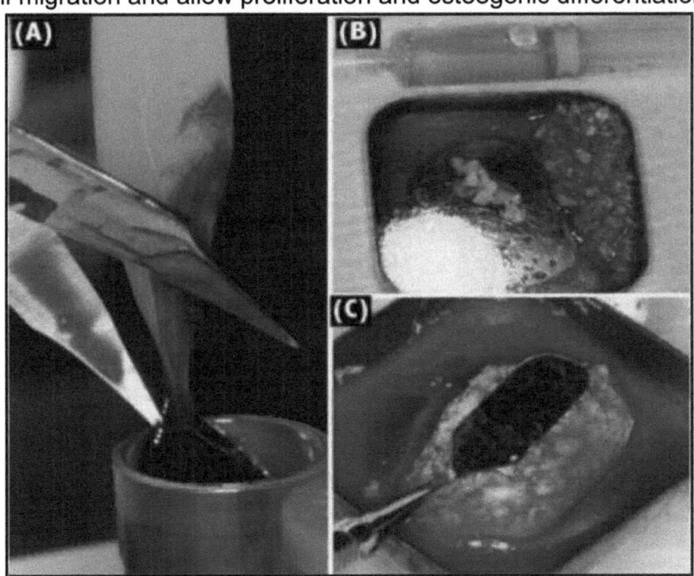

Figure 13. The sequence of the protocol to obtain composite PRF/particulate xenograft: (A) Extraction of PRF membranes from tubes; (B) Irrigation of autologous bone and xenograft with liquid fibrinogen; (C) Obtaining composite particulate PRF/xenograft. (23)

4.1.2.3. Maintaining space for bone neoformation

Maintaining the scar space is based on the biological principles of ROG, and is a crucial factor in the success of guided bone regeneration procedures, in order to allow bone neoformation to take place under optimum conditions and achieve the expected results, enabling the implant to be positioned correctly. The PTFE membranes reinforced with titanium and the slow resorption time of the filling materials help to maintain the scar space.

Furthermore, the anatomy of the bone defect can ë1re sometimes favourable for maintaining the space and preventing the membrane from collapsing. When the geometry of the defect is concave, with 3 walls, it will be suitable for maintaining the stability of the membrane and will therefore help to preserve the scar space.

When they cannot maintain the space, another technique is applied:

Space maintenance using the tenting screw (24) The advantage of the tenting screw technique is its ability to create space. During the healing period, diagonally placed tenting screws provide a tenting effect and resist membrane collapse by maintaining the volume and geometry of the space.

The advantages of this technique are

- Ease of use.
- Provides space for the growth of osteogenic cells.
- Low morbidity.
- Shorter healing time.
- Economical.

Osteosynthesis screws are made of titanium and are available in several lengths: 6, 8, 10 and 12 mm and in several diameters: from 1.4 to 2.0 mm.

Tentation screws are used as follows: The osteotomy for the tent screw is prepared before the screw is placed, using a mini-mill. By appropriately plating titanium temptation screws surrounded by allografts and covered with resorbable membranes, it is possible to augment major crestal defects without harvesting autogenous bone. The result is very favourable, allowing safe osteogenesis and restoration of the horizontal height of the bone crests.

The overall success of this procedure depends on the appropriate design of the tissue flaps and tension-free primary closure.

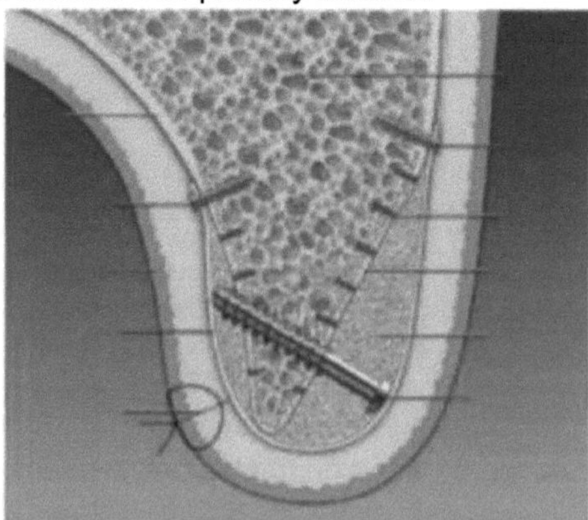

Figure 14. Space maintenance using the tent screw technique (24)

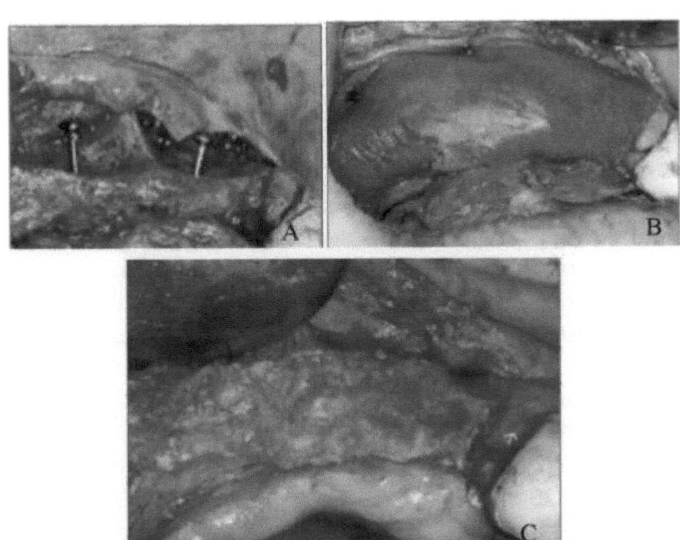

Figure 15. A and B: use of tent screws + lyophilised demineralised bone + bioresorbable membrane on a 2 mm wide crete; C: re-entry after 6 months: presence of a significant increase in bone volume, the width of the crete is 7 to 8 mm (24).

4.1.3.   ROG operating protocol

Several factors can influence the result of horizontal bone gain by ROG, such as the regeneration technique, incision design, flap management, preparation of the recipient site, establishing graft stability and tension-free primary closure. To achieve this, the practitioner must be well equipped during the surgical stage of the ROG.

4.1.3.1.   Pre-implant ROG (14)

The surgical procedure is carried out in accordance with high standards of surgical hygiene in order to reduce the risk of contamination by extra-oral bacteria. The peribuccal skin is disinfected with an anti-septic solution and the mouth is rinsed with a chlorhexidine solution.

- **Anaesthesia** will be administered in the conventional way, using periapical injections or locoregional injections in the posterior region.
- Slightly palatal/lingual **crestal incision** to be made at a distance from the site to be regenerated.
- Full thickness **detachment of the mucosa** to gain access to the cortices. This detachment becomes partial when apical to the defect, in order to guarantee the elasticity of the flap for subsequent closure without any tension.
- The granulation tissue and fibrous tissue are **debrided** to prepare the site for correct positioning of the filling material and membranes.
- **Passivation of the flap through a periosteal incision** to ensure primary closure of the site
- **Drilling and fixation of osteosynthesis screws using tent pegs** (if this

technique has been indicated): drilling is carried out using a hand-piece drill.

• The bone is **decorticated** by perforations within the crete to provide endosteal stimulation, stimulating angiogenesis and releasing growth factors to promote healing.

• **The placement of the biomaterial** within the space dedicated to bone regeneration after its preparation.

• **The membrane** is cut at **the top** without sharp angles (to avoid damaging the mucous membrane) and must be pressed tightly against the biomaterial below. Its dimensions must be sufficient on each side (3mm minimum) to hold the biomaterial particles in place. It must therefore be placed at a distance from the incisions to avoid the risk of subsequent exposure. Likewise, it should be kept away from teeth, which could lead to infectious contamination.

• **Membrane fixation:** using pins or periosteal sutures.

• **Repositioning the flap:** the flap must completely cover the membrane to minimise the risk of exposure.

• Hermetic suturing using discontinuous stitches, without creating tension.

• Post-operative prescription: mouthwash + paracetamol + amoxicillin-based antibiotic for 6 days to avoid any complications.

• Advise the patient not to brush the surgical site and to use chlorhexidine digluconate rinses twice a day for plaque control.

4.1.3.2.   Per-implant ROG (18)

The special feature is that the ROG elements will be positioned on the exposed surface of the implant. Once the site of the future implant has been exposed, the operating protocol is as follows:

• Selection of the right type of implant (length and diameter)

• Drilling and placement of the implant, respecting the distances of
safety and the prothetic project axis.

• Filling biomaterial after treatment
directly on the exposed surface of the implant.

• Application of the membrane on top, which must be in intimate contact with the biomaterial. The membrane will be cut into 2 pieces, one smaller and one larger, and these will then be placed using a double layer technique.

A technique has been described for the purpose of guided bone regeneration per-implant: this is the bone augmentation technique using a two-layer composite graft and a collagen membrane. It consists of applying 2 filling materials of different origins in 2 layers to the exposed part of the implant. The first layer will be in direct contact with the implant, and is made up of fragments of autogenous bone taken locally from the anterior nasal spine and kept in a solution containing the patient's collected blood mixed with a sterile isotonic sodium chloride solution (0.5%) or a Ringer's solution (0.9%) to prevent coagulation. After a certain amount of time (15 to 20 minutes), this mixture releases several growth factors known as BCM (bone-conditioned medium).

The second layer on top consists of particles of deproteinated bovine bone mineral soaked in the BCM solution, which is rich in growth factors that biologically activate the bovine bone particles. The composite graft is then covered with a non-reticulated collagen membrane moistened with BCM solution, also cut into 2 pieces and applied in 2 double layers.

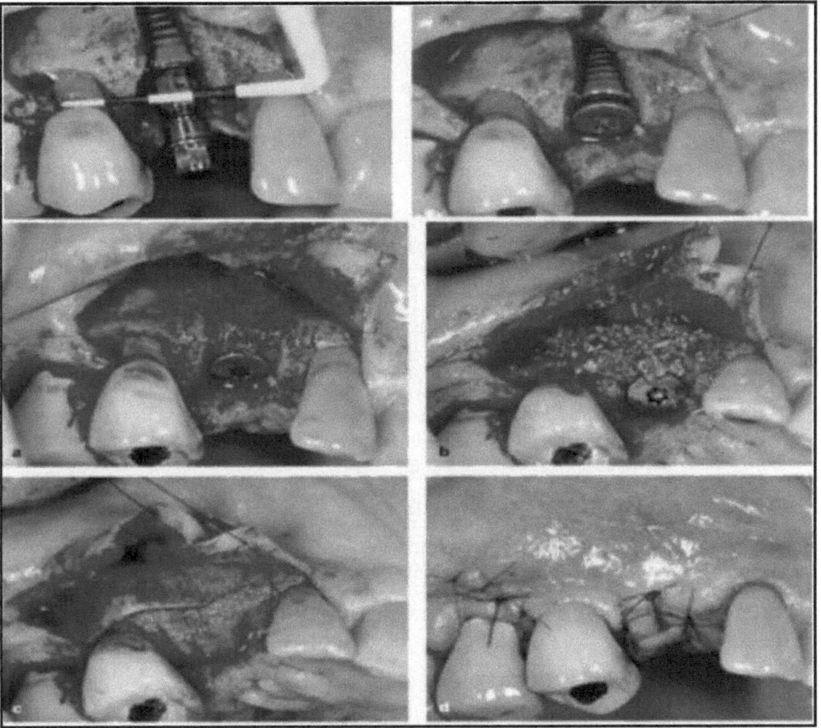

Figure 16. Operating protocol for per-implant guided bone regeneration at site la 13 with a horizontal bone defect (18)

Another technique that can be applied per-implant when the defect has a single wall bone morphology is the sausage technique. Urban et al originally described this method, which can be used in cases where the implant surface is level with the buccal bone surface or slightly outside the bone socket. This technique uses a collagen membrane fixed by titanium pins. The aim is to stabilise the filling material on the bone so that there is no migration or collapse of the particles (18).

4.1.4. Choice of protocol depending on the morphology of the bone defect

The surgical approach to ROG also depends on the morphology of the defect at the implant site. The number of bone walls has an impact on the potential for bone neoformation at the pre- or peri-implant site.

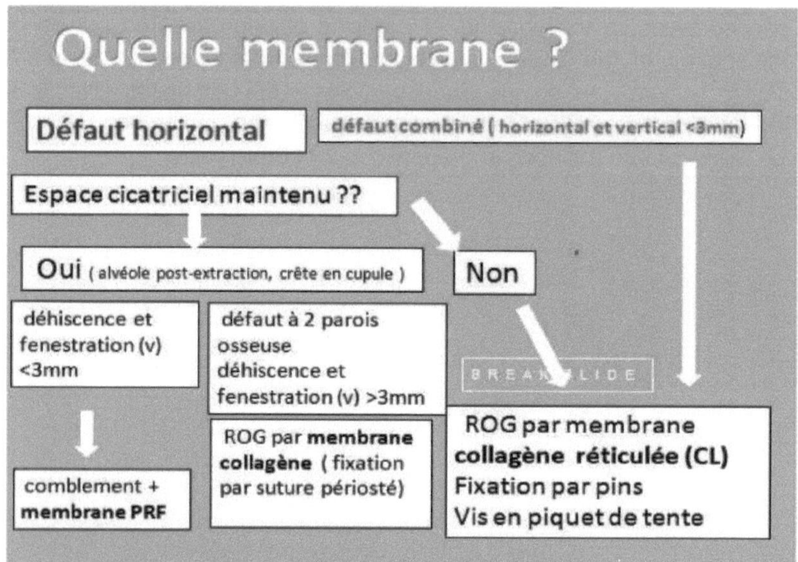

Figure 17. Representative diagram of surgical procedures according to defect morphology (18)

4.2. Autogenous bone grafting

4.2.1. Definition and interest

According to Maujean et al (2003), appositional bone grafts refer to the surgical procedure of bringing material in the form of autogenous screwed bone blocks to a site containing vertical or horizontal bone insufficiency with the aim of restoring bone structure and thus achieving implant stability.

autogenous screwed bone blocks to a site containing vertical or horizontal bone insufficiency with the aim of restoring bone structure and thus achieving implant stability. (8)

4.2.2.　　Origin of the graft

The combination of the onlay grafting procedure with autogenous bone material makes it possible to increase bone thickness in extremely resorbed maxillae (Chiapasco et al. 1998; Nystrom et al. 2004).

Table VI. Representative table of the advantages and disadvantages of the autogenous graft

Autogenous graft

Advantages -	Disadvantages
The only one with osteogenic properties (osteogenic cells from cancellous bone) - Osteoinductive, osteoconductive. - Biocompatibility. - Promotes angiogenesis and rapid healing. - Donor sites provide a high cell survival rate, a high concentration of growth factors, and are embryologically similar to buccal recipient sites. - Reduced risk of resorption - Minimal risk of rejection or transmission of infectious diseases. - A single surgical procedure. - Reasonable cost	- The volume of intra-oral samples is limited. - The need for a second practitioner for extra-oral harvesting. - Adapting the graft to the shape of the donor site is a little tricky, leading to a relatively long surgical time. - The creation of a second surgical site leads to post-operative complications. - The skill of the practitioner is essential, a technique reserved for oral surgeons.

At the time, extra-oral sampling from the iliac crest and ribs was commonly used. However, their use was restricted due to a number of disadvantages such as intense and disabling postoperative pain. According to Younger and Chapman (1989), 8.6% of patients experienced post-operative complications after extra-oral sampling, such as infection, bleeding and pain. Resorption was also significant post-operatively (Adell et al., 1990; Widmark, 2001), with a variation in final volume of up to 50% (Johansson et al., 2001).

To overcome these drawbacks, we opted for cranial rather than iliac specimens. The reason for this decision is that the post-operative period is less demanding and the scar is virtually invisible. In addition, it would appear that post-operative resorption is significantly lower with flat skull bones due to their membranous origin. This characteristic could favour more rapid revascularisation than with bones of euchondral origin(25).

Table VII. Comparison of extra-oral sampling sites (3)

Origin	Benefits	Disadvantages
Parietal bone	- Same embryonic origin - less resorption - The proximity of the sites	- 2 operating sites. - Morbidity - surgery under general anaesthetic - graft quantity limit

Iliac bone	- Large amount of bone - good bone density (cortico-spongiosa)	- Post-operative resorption - post-operative complications (pain, redemptions, etc.) - need for 2 practitioners (2 operating sites)

Because of its many advantages, cranial bone remains the undisputed reference for maxillary apposition grafts. However, in order to compensate for the inconvenience of extra-oral harvesting, intra-oral harvesting sites such as the chin symphysis and ramus have also been proposed. These sites offer a promising alternative, providing satisfactory aesthetic and functional results. In addition, these samples can be taken easily by a single practitioner and do not require general anaesthesia. (25)

Mandibular bone grafts, which are mainly made from cortical bone, have low volume loss and excellent incorporation with short healing times. However, the amount of bone they can provide is only sufficient to correct small to medium bone defects. (25)

- **Graft of symphyseal origin :**

In 2000, Montazem and colleagues conducted a study to determine the maximum amount of cortico-cancellous bone that could be removed from the symphysis without compromising the integrity of the chin nerve, its incisal extension, the roots of the front teeth or the bone profile. Their research, based on the analysis of 16 cadavers, showed that the average size of the bone blocks removed was 21 x 9.9 x 6.9 mm, ranging from a minimum of 21 x 6.5 x 6 mm to a maximum of 25 x 13 x 9 mm. This patient-dependent quantity of bone can correct a bone defect involving two to three teeth. (25)

In addition, this type of graft is characterised by good bone quality due to the high density of the chin symphysis. In addition, the harvesting technique is considered easier than for other donor sites, due to the ease of surgical access at this level.

These specimens must be taken from either side of the mid-chin area, in order to preserve the aesthetics of the patient's profile and not to cause any changes to the patient's profile. The wound is then closed using sutures in 2 planes: the muscular plane and the mucosal plane.

However, it is possible to encounter certain common post-operative complications after this type of extraction, such as redemas, significant pain and altered incisal sensitivity. These risks have led a number of authors to favour the use of root canal harvesting.

- **Graft of ramic origin: (26)**

Many clinicians have concluded that the ramus region offers several advantages over other donor sites for bone augmentation techniques. In fact, this donor site is generally characterised by thick cortical tissue surrounding good quality cancellous tissue. Moreover, ramus harvesting no longer alters the patient's aesthetics, while causing less sensory disturbance or post-operative discomfort than symphyseal harvesting.

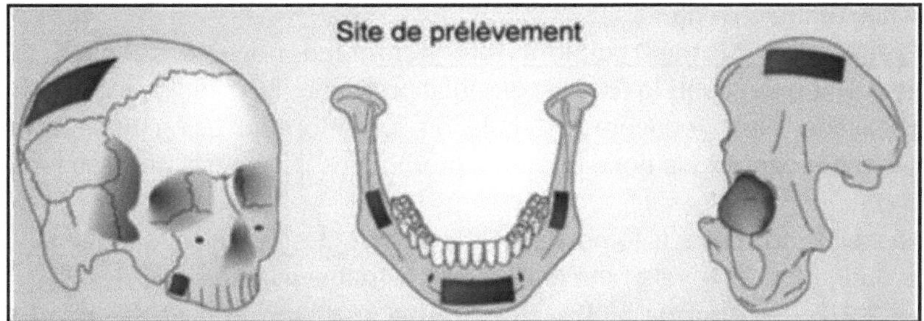

Figure 18. Intra-oral and extra-oral sampling sites. (14)

However, the anatomical limits of the ramus, such as the coronoid process, the molars, the inferior alveolar canal and the width of the posterior mandible, must be taken into consideration. If the inferior alveolar canal is positioned upwards in relation to the external oblique crete, or if the width of the ramus is less than 1 cm, other donor sites should be considered. Similarly, limited opening of the mandible, temporomandibular joint dysfunction and compromised clinical access may complicate bone harvesting. Specific pathologies such as pericoronitis or other pathologies associated with an impacted third molar and a history of sagittal mandibular osteotomy may contraindicate bone harvesting in this region. In addition, post-operative complications are still valid, such as: gënant trismus, dysesthesia and paresthesia due to lesion of the inferior alveolar nerve during the operation.

4.2.3. Operating protocol

Surgery is performed in several stages:
- Incision and exposure of the recipient site
- Harvesting the graft from the donor site
- Adjusting and stabilising the graft at the recipient site: this is a crucial stage that determines the success of the operation.

4.2.3.1.   Preparation of the recipient site

1.   Local anaesthetic The procedure begins with the generous administration of an anaesthetic to the juxta-periosteum and para-apical region, on both the vestibular and palatal/lingual sides.

2.   Incision: The incision is made at the top of the crete, with a slight displacement in the palatal region. It is then followed by vertical offloading, which must be away from the site to optimise vascularisation.

3.   Flap detachment: involves detaching the flap from the full thickness. At this stage, the recipient site must be clearly visible so that it can be analysed and a graft adapted to the specific bone defect can be harvested. In the case of a posterior mandibular graft, it is essential to passivate the flap on the floor side by dissecting the superficial fibres of the mylohyoid muscle. When dissecting the flap on the vestibular side, care must be taken not to lesion the branches of the chin nerve.

4. **Preparation of the recipient site itself**: the bone is debrided using curettes and ultrasound to remove granulation tissue, followed by washing with chlorhexidine. Next, endosteal stimulation is performed using bone burs to stimulate the cancellous bone and thus promote osteogenesis and subsequent healing.

It is possible to make a template of the recipient site which will serve as a guide during the removal of the graft identical to the situation.

4.2.3.2.　Access to the donor site and removal of the graft

There are 2 possible incisions at the symphyseal level:

• A sulcular incision is followed by vertical cuts distal to the first molars, allowing clear visualization of the chin foramina.

However, this incision pattern is not valid for the thin gingival biotype because of the risk of recession that it can cause post-operatively.

• A V-shaped incision is made in the symphyseal region along the mucogingival line of the mandibular canines, followed by one or two small cuts, taking care not to loosen the mucogingival branch close to the canine (14).

For the ramus, the incision starts at the vestibule, from the anterior edge of the ascending ramus (not higher than the occlusal plane to avoid lesion of the buccal artery or exposure of the fatty body of the cheek), medially to the external oblique ridge and continues anteriorly and laterally, parallel to this line, to the distal aspect of the 2nd mandibular premolar. (26)

Tracing the osteotomy and harvesting the graft: the trace of the osteotomy is initially marked by regular perforations of the bone cortex. These holes are then connected using a tapered fissure burr inserted into a handpiece or disc, under continuous irrigation. There are special semi-lunar ramus harvesting discs with vestibular protection (Dr Zastrow's kit). It is also possible to use inserts or an angled saw on piezotomes.

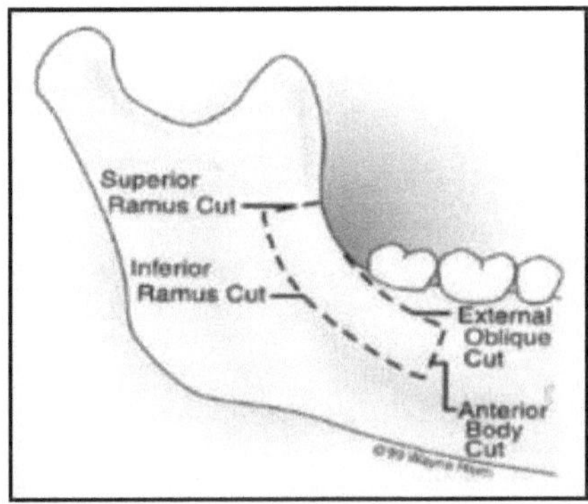

Figure 19. Schematic presentation of the four osteotomies for harvesting ramus bone(26)

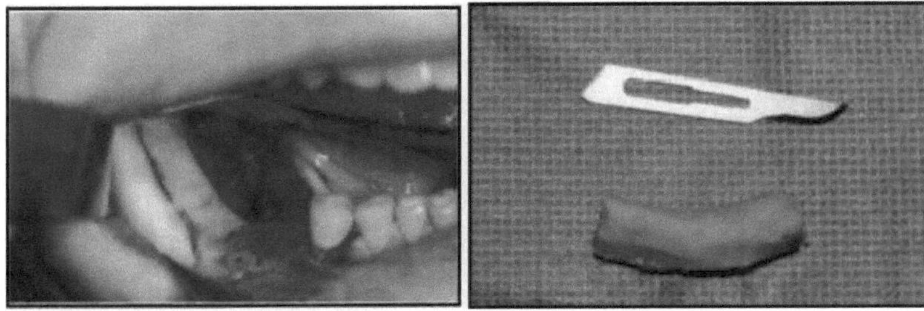

Figure 20. Ramic graft removal (26)

After the fenêtre has been created, the graft is then harvested either using piezotome inserts or a surgical mallet is used to percuss a bone chisel to loosen the graft, while holding the mandible firmly.

It is important that the graft is thick enough to envelop the vestibular cortex, which is often important at both chin and ramus level, as well as the internal cancellous bone.

It should be noted that the harvested piece must be slightly oversized to allow fagging adapted to the recipient site, but care must be taken not to compromise the integrity of the dental roots or the lingual cortex, in order to avoid any fracture of the mandible.

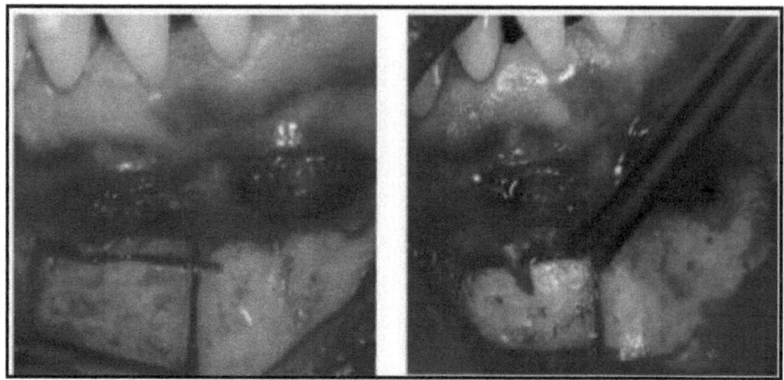
Figure 21. Osteotomy tracing and removal of the symphyseal graft (14)

For the symphyseal harvest, safety distances must be respected during the manoeuvre: 3mm from the dental roots; 5mm from the mandibular foramen; 5mm from the basilar edge. In addition, it is recommended that the medial osteotomy line be positioned 2mm from the symphyseal midline. Alfred Sebban also recommends taking two small lateral samples rather than a single medial one, in order to preserve the patient's facial structure.

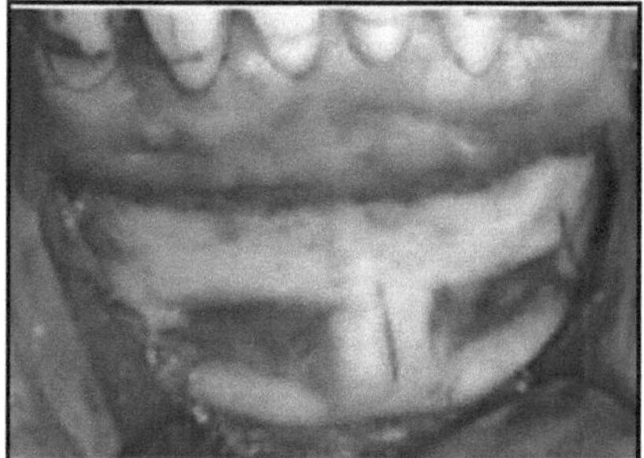
Figure 22. Para-symphyseal sampling(14)

Once the graft has been harvested, immediate attention must be paid to softening and adapting the graft en bloc to the recipient site. The graft can be preserved in sterile physiological serum if necessary. No attempt should be made to harvest additional cancellous bone from the donor site. A hemostatic dressing (collagen, gelatin sponge, oxidised regenerated cellulose, PRF) can be placed in the donor area if required. Site closure can be achieved after graft fixation and suturing of the recipient site with a continuous suture.

There are several surgical techniques for obtaining a stable bone graft at the recipient site, which favours osteogenesis and correction of the horizontal bone defect and therefore allows optimal integration of the implant, such as :

• Block grafting or onlay grafting
• Form-facing grafting

4.2.3.3.   Block graft or onlay graft (28) (14)

As its name suggests, this technique uses a graft in the form of a cortico-cancellous block without any major modification of the graft.

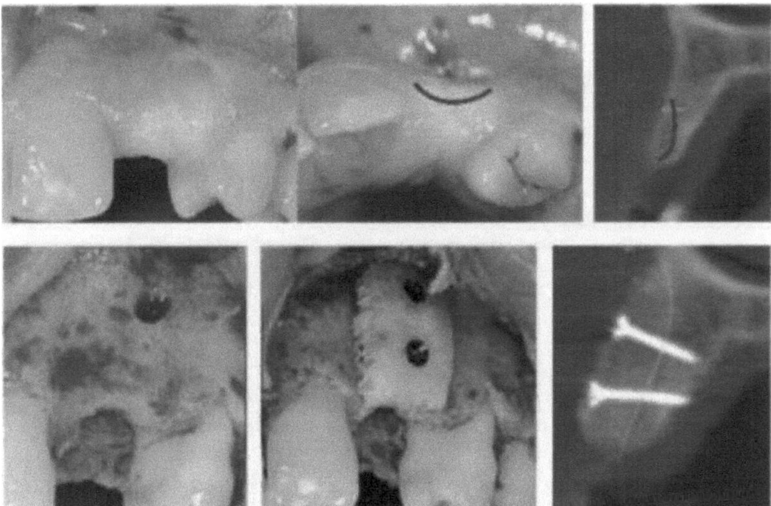
Figure 23. Placement of an autogenous bone block (14)

Onlay grafting is mainly indicated in the maxilla because of the cancellous bone quality, which allows easy revascularisation of the cortico-cancellous block. In the mandible, the cortical bone is generally thick, making it difficult to revascularise the large block, which leads to its resorption. In addition, the block is exposed to several muscular and ligament insertions in the mandible, which affects the stability of the graft.

To prevent post-operative infections, we recommend antibiotic therapy (Augmentin for 7 days) and daily rinsing with mouthwash for 1 to 2 weeks.

However, given the problems of revascularisation of the graft and the horizontal increase limited to the width of the graft, this technique is increasingly being abandoned in favour of formwork techniques.

4.2.3.4. Form-facing graft (27)

Formwork grafting, described by F. Khoury, is currently the reference technique that we prefer to use, particularly on narrow alveolar crates.

It consists of dividing the graft into 2 parts as follows: the cortical bone is separated from the cancellous bone which will be placed and fixed using osteosynthesis screws opposite the bone defect, being the lateral wall of the crate, to serve as a support for the filling material, this inter-cortical space determines the quantity of bone to be regenerated. Secondly, the cancellous bone of the graft is ground into bone chips using a bone mill, which then fills the inter-cortical space already created.

After the graft has been harvested, it is thinned to allow it to be positioned at the recipient site as a thin lateral wall of the reconstruction, while retaining enough strength to be fixed with screws (less than 1mm thick). The thinned cortex then becomes more revascularisable than the initial cortex, which reduces the risk of long-term resorption. In addition, refining the graft using a bone scraper allows a generous quantity of bone chips to be collected and used to fill the space to be regenerated (Figure 54).

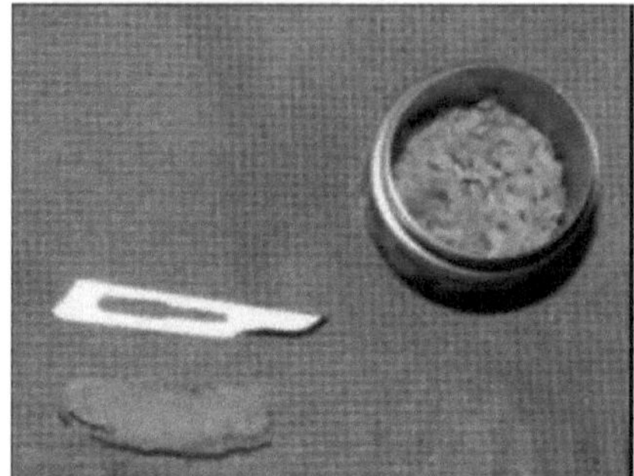

Figure 24. Thinned cortex and bone chips collected after grinding (27)

A slice is then made apically in relation to the defect to be regenerated, allowing the graft cortex to be positioned correctly.

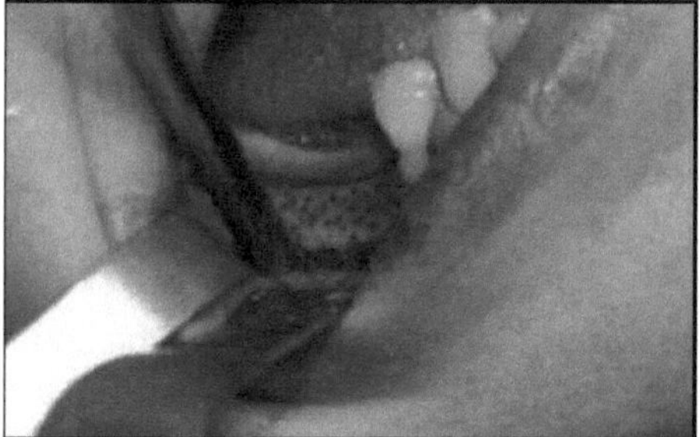

Figure 25. Slicing (under surgical suction) for graft fixation (27)

Before positioning the graft, perforations should be made in the graft bed to encourage neovascularisation of the bone particles and stimulate osteogenesis.
Correct positioning of the graft cortex stabilises the internal bone chips and the blood clot, acting as a barrier to soft tissue growth, thereby promoting healing and bone re-formation.

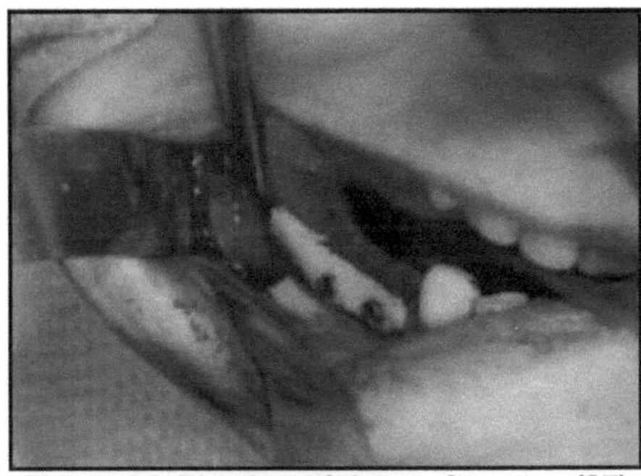
Figure 26. Fixation of the graft cortex (27)

In the case of a heavily resorbed crete in both the horizontal and vertical directions, it is possible to correct the bone deficiency in both directions at the same time using the double formwork technique using both vestibular and lingual cortices.

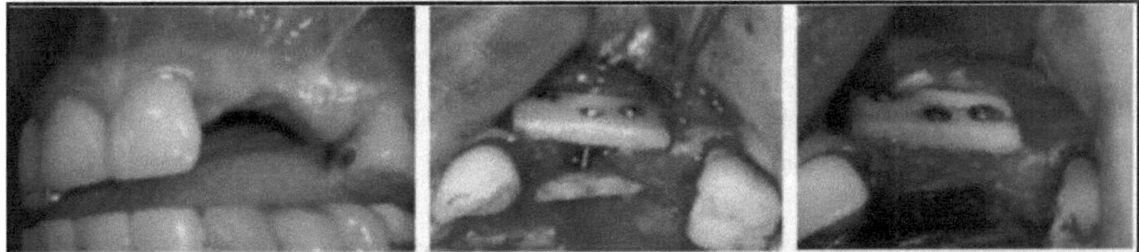
Figure 27. Double formwork technique to correct a combined defect (14)

4.2.4. Next steps
4.2.4.1.   Healing
Regardless of the grafting technique adopted, the healing time is relatively short, varying between 4 and 6 months. Implant placement is only indicated when the control cone beam shows complete bone regeneration of the defect. Subsequent implant healing times are based on the healing quality of the graft site, which generally results in a healing phase of 4 to 6 months. In addition, the implant placed after the time allowed for complete ossification shows good primary stability due to the good bone quality offered by the apposition graft. (29)

The apposition graft provides a generous amount of neoformed bone up to 7 mm wide.

Similarly for the donor site, complete healing at this level takes relatively 4 months.

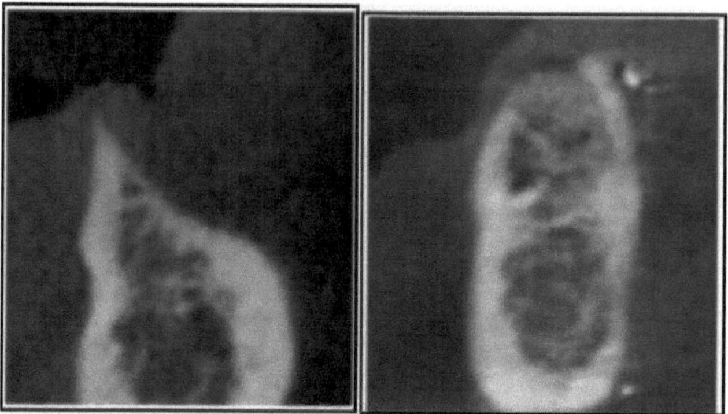

Figure 28. Complete bone neoformation 4 months after form-fit grafting (27)

The radiological signs of graft success are :
- The fusion of the cortical bone with that of the residual crete.
- Bone formation in harmony with native bone.
- Missing radiocards.

4.2.4.2.   Possible complications

- The most common and damaging complication associated with bone grafts is wound dehiscence and bone exposure during healing. This is most often due to inadequate manipulation of the flap and a lack of tension-free soft tissue closure.
- The risk of graft resorption varies between 25% and 50% during the first 6 months. Some authors recommend over-correcting the bone defect as a precautionary measure.
- Post-operative infections at the recipient site cause partial or total graft failure.
- Post-operative pain and redemas at the donor sites.
- Risk of dysaesthesia and paraesthesia in the region of the donor sites following lesion of the nerve structures during harvesting.

4.3. Transverse bone expansion

4.3.1.   Definition

The method of alveolar crete expansion was originally developed by Dr Hilt Tatum in the 1970s and was commonly referred to as the crete division technique, bone spreading or crete expansion.

Its aim is to encourage bone formation around the implant sites by creating bony osteotomies that allow the buccal cortex to be repositioned after a green stick fracture of the buccal bone wall. Since its introduction, numerous studies have been conducted to demonstrate that the alveolar crete division technique is an effective alternative to traditional horizontal alveolar augmentation procedures. (30)

4.3.2. Characteristics of a crete candidate for crestal expansion

The bone expansion technique is not always applicable to horizontal bone defects. A number of conditions must be met at the level of the residual defect for this technique to be used correctly:

• A minimum thickness of 3 mm, allowing an osteotomy to be performed without damaging the cortices.

• An adequate crest height of at least 7mm is available.

• The cortices must be sufficiently thin to provide a degree of malleability to facilitate expansion and reduce the risk of fracture.

• The walls must be convergent and parallel after expansion.

• An articular reverse of no more than 3 mm, which allows an ideal inter-arch relationship to be achieved after the operation.

• A crestal orientation favourable to osteotomy traction. (14)

4.3.3. Operating protocol

The operating protocol for this technique differs depending on the arch, due to the difference in bone density in each arch. In the maxilla, expansion is performed in a single surgical step, and bone expansion and implant placement can be performed simultaneously. In the mandible, the operation is performed in 2 stages in order to prevent cortical fracture. (31)(32)

Preoperatively, it is essential to assess the alveolar ridge visually and by palpation. Palpating the ridge with two fingers and sliding them along the ridge gives a tactile sensation of its thinness, as well as detecting the presence of bony undercuts(31).

There are 2 possible surgical procedures:

• Bone splitting" expansion of the crete

• Bone spreading" expansion of the crete by dilation

We will now describe the bone spreading technique used to treat the 2nd clinical case.

4.3.3.1. Bone spreading (33)

The spreading technique is an alternative to the Summers osteotome method and uses specially tapered screws or spacers to exert lateral compression on the bone and increase the density of the cancellous region adjacent to the site. This spacer allows controlled and standardised dilatation of the horizontal bone. This technique involves horizontal bone augmentation with minimal trauma for simultaneous implant placement.

One of the main advantages of the crestal expansion technique is that it is less invasive. This technique allows the density of the jawbone to be reinforced, which promotes greater initial implant stability.

The surgical technique begins with a crestal incision, followed by the detachment of a full-thickness flap to expose the alveolar crete. However, some authors recommend the use of partial thickness flaps for blood supply and periosteal vascularisation, which ensures the vitality of the displaced segment. In fact, the revascularisation of the displaced segment no longer comes from the internal cancellous bone, as with other bone augmentation techniques, but rather from the external periosteum. The periosteum plays an essential role in the vascularisation of the separated cortex and in osteogenesis within the subsequent site. Gray et al concluded that at least a third of osteogenesis could be attributed to the periosteum alone. However, complete detachment of a full-thickness flap results in the removal of the periosteal vascular pedicle from the vestibular cortex, leading to the formation of a devascularised free fragment, which induces resorption.

Next, the sites to be implanted were marked using an initial burr rotating at 18,000 rpm, while benefiting from generous irrigation with sterile saline solution, which allowed the cortical plate to be extracted. The use of this burr thus prevents the following instrument from derapping.

The pilot drill is then introduced, creating a sub-dimensional bone cavity (smaller than normal) that reaches the desired depth.

This is followed by a successive pass of a series of spreaders (the order of diameter and coding of the instruments must be respected) (figure), taking care to advance as slowly as possible. The spreaders must be carefully screwed on using a suitable conveyor and, if necessary, the driver.

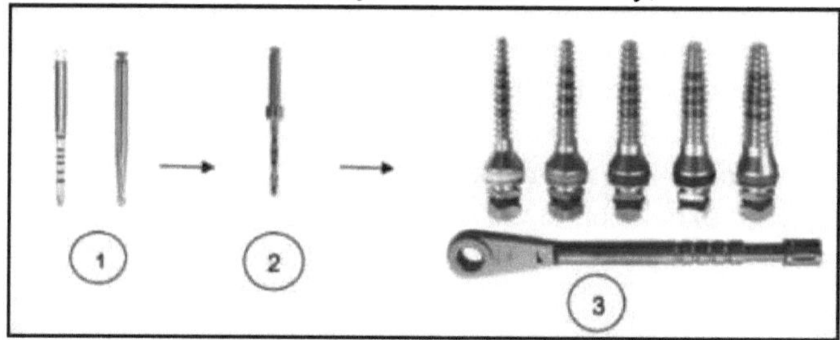

Figure 29. The sequence of spreaders used to expand the ridge (14)

With each insertion of a larger expander, the bone is shifted laterally until the desired width is achieved. The implant must be slightly larger in diameter than the site created by the last expander.

At the end of this procedure, the flaps are hermetically sutured in their original position.

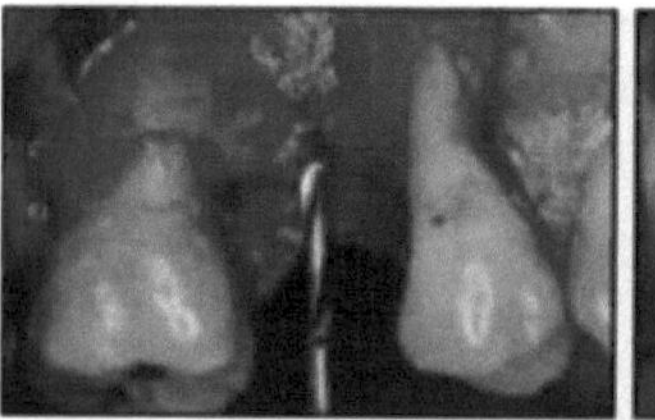
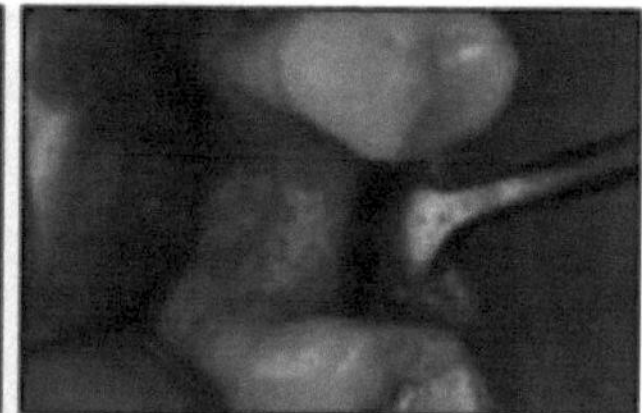

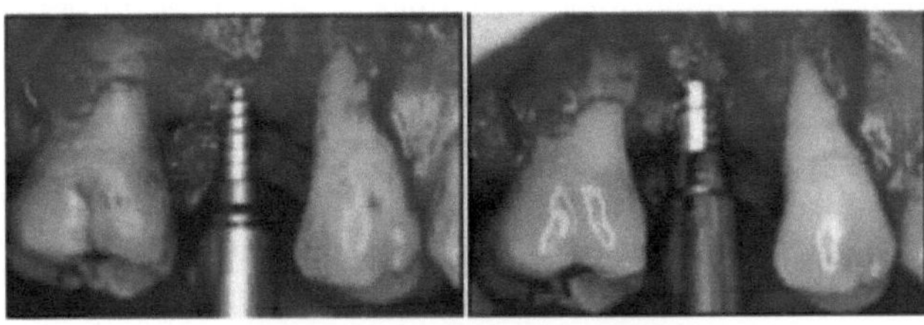

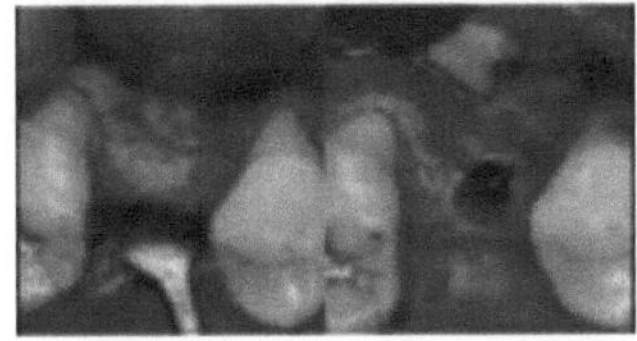

Figure 30. Sequence of the surgical procedure for crete dilatation (33)

A 7-day course of antibiotics and analgesics is recommended to prevent any possible post-operative complications.

Patients should be advised not to rinse their mouths vigorously and to use ice packs on the surgical area for the first 24 hours after the operation.

4.3.4.   Post-operative care

Horizontal bone expansion can result in an average bone volume gain of 5 mm or more, depending on the technique used. Research carried out on 6 patients who had undergone bone expansion showed a bone increase ranging from 5.6 to 7.33 mm (34).

By using a two-stage crete procedure, the width of the crete can be doubled or even tripled (31).

The enlarged bone void can sometimes reach a thickness of 9 mm. However, it is crucial to take into account possible bone resorption, which can lead to a reduction of a few millimetres in the volume gained (on average 1.5 mm). Consequently, the crete may have a volume of 7 mm after the operation. (14)

This procedure is less prone to resorption and infectious complications. Admittedly, the 2-stage surgical approach reduces possible post-operative complications and provides a more stable long-term result. (30) (31)

In addition, piezosurgery is more effective in expanding bone during the early stages of bone healing. This method leads to a more anticipated increase in bone morphogenetic proteins, provides better control of the inflammatory process and stimulates osteogenesis (34).

4.3.5.   Comparison with other augmentation techniques (35) (36)

The dividing crete technique offers significant advantages in terms of augmentation. In fact, it reduces the treatment time compared with traditional bone grafting methods, as it does not require a bone healing period of 4 to 6 months before placing the implant. In addition, it minimises complications by avoiding the need for a second surgical site for bone harvesting, which causes a number of intra- and post-operative problems such as unpredictable resorption of the autogenous graft material, prolonged treatment time for the patient due to a healing period for the autogenous graft, risks of damage to the vascular and neural structures generated during harvesting, and the possibility of exposure of the graft.

In addition, this approach appears to be less aggressive and less invasive than other techniques such as autogenous apposition grafting.

A comparative study between the split-crete technique and autogenous bone block grafting revealed no significant difference in implant survival between the two treatment modalities. Similarly, the amount of bone regenerated by these 2 approaches appears to be similar.

However, it is important to note that the indications for the crete expansion technique require a minimum horizontal crete width of around 3 mm.

It is also necessary to use a partial thickness flap, especially for the bone splitting expansion technique, in order to preserve the periosteal vascularisation of the vestibular fragment and avoid its resorption, which may constitute an additional difficulty making the operative protocol dependent.

In addition, mandibular alveolar deficits with a lack of elasticity, high cortical density or proximity to the external oblique line in the posterior region of the mandible hinder the mobility and expansion of the cortical crevices.

However, in the case of severe alveolar deficits accompanied by thick cortical bone plates, the outcome of treatment after a divided cruciate may be compromised. This is because intervention of the cancellous bone layer is necessary to facilitate the use of instruments to expand the alveolar crete and ensure adequate blood supply during the healing phase.

5.
CLINICAL CASES OF AUGMENTATION HORIZONTAL

5. CLINICAL CASES OF HORIZONTAL AUGMENTATION

5.1. Clinical case N°1

Patient S.F, aged 30, in good general health, consulted the dental medicine department of the Farhat Hached University Hospital in Sousse, for implant-supported rehabilitation of teeth 11 and 12, which had been extracted following coronal-radicular fractures caused by an old trauma.

Clinical examination of the anterior site reveals :

- The clinical absence of 11 and 12.
- a straight, thin, indented ridge in the horizontal direction with a vestibular depression perceptible on palpation.
- Insufficient hygiene.
- A thick periodontal biotype.

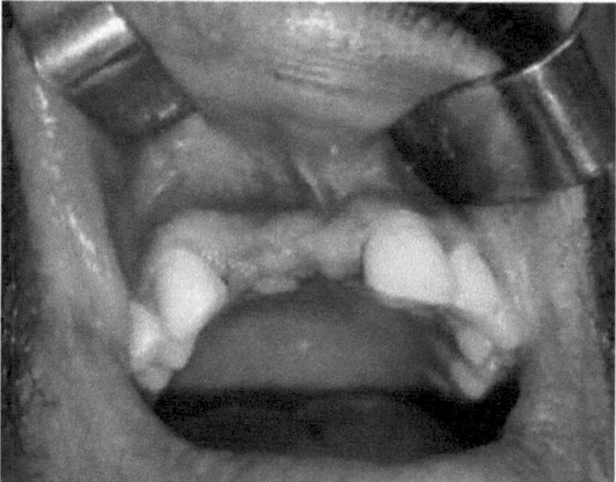

Figure 31. Endo-buccal view showing the absence of 11 and 12

Radiological examination :

An examination of the maxillary cone beam was carried out: the oblique coronal sections passing through the edentulous sector revealed a severe horizontal bone defect at the sites of 11 and 12.

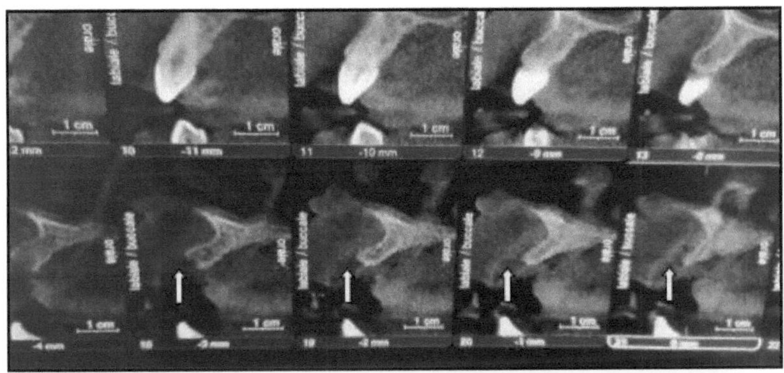

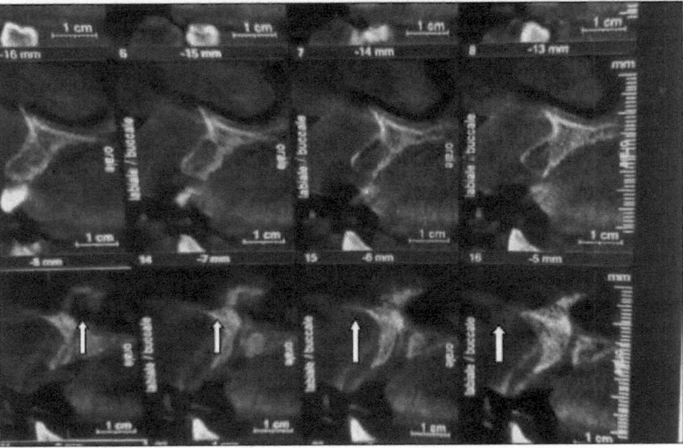

Figure 32. Oblique coronal sections through the sites of 11 and 12 showing horizontal volume insufficiency with a 3mm wide crevice.

Therapeutic decision :

Implant-supported rehabilitation of 11 and 12 with an autogenous casing graft using a symphyseal pre-implant harvest to correct the horizontal bone defect.

Operating protocol :

The steps in the operating protocol are illustrated in the following figures:

 **Pre-implant graft :**

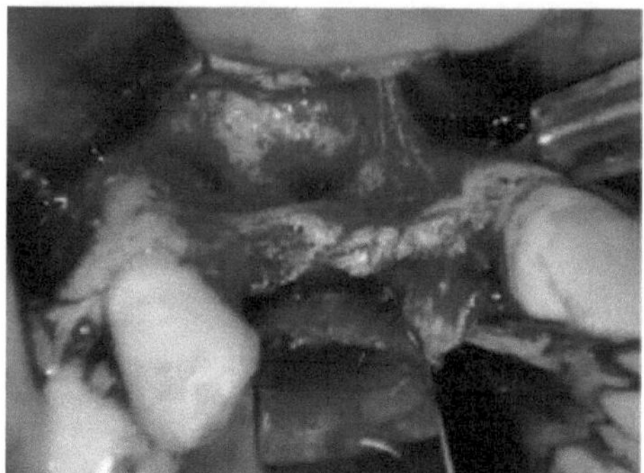

Figure 33. After anaesthesia, an incision is made, followed by detachment of the flap in the full thickness of the recipient site, to reveal the horizontal bone defect.

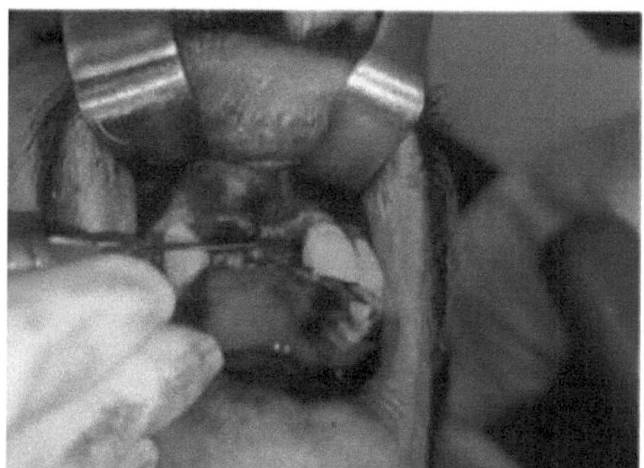

Figure 34. Debridement of granulation and fibrous tissue, endosteal stimulation and intraoperative verification of graft size.

❖ Symphyseal sampling:

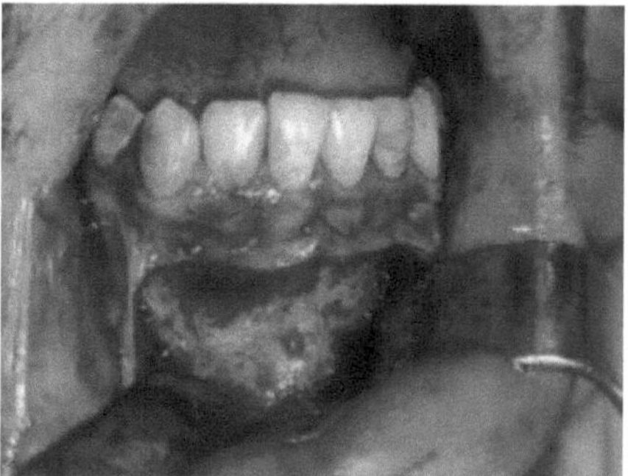

Figure 35. After anaesthesia, an incision was made at the base of the vestibule, 5 mm beyond the muco-gingival line running from canine to canine, and the flap was detached by freeing the muscle attachments in the chin region.

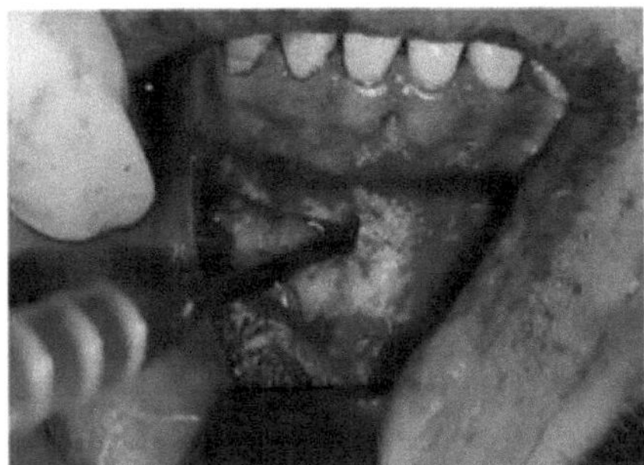

Figure 36. After piezosurgery of the osteotomy tracing, dislocation and graft harvesting, the PRF was placed (in order to reduce postoperative complications).

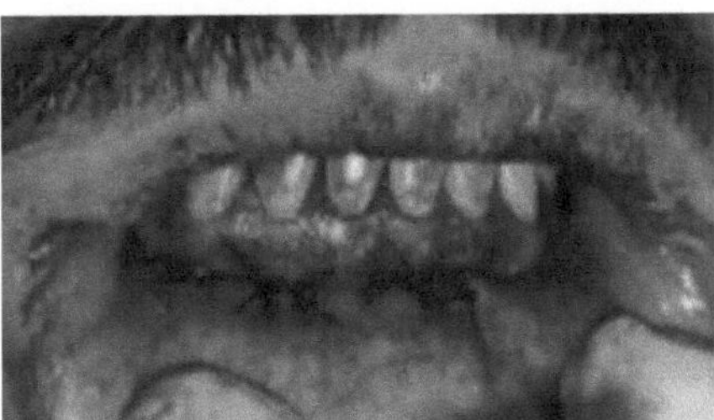

Figure 37. Closure of the wound using separating and hermetic sutures (sutures made in 2 planes: muscular and mucosal)

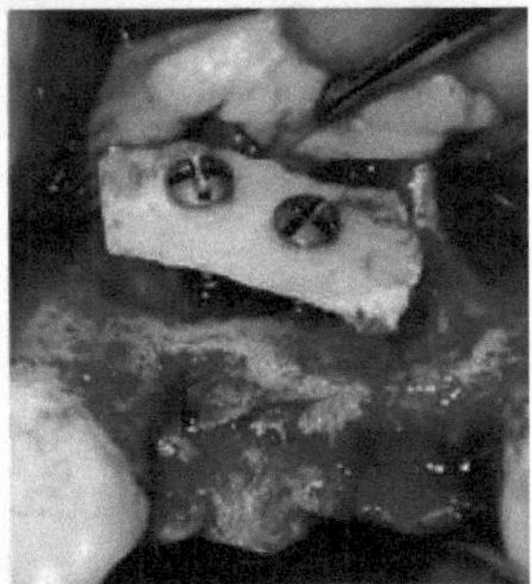

Figure 38. Adaptation and fixation of the cortical graft using 2 osteosynthesis screws.

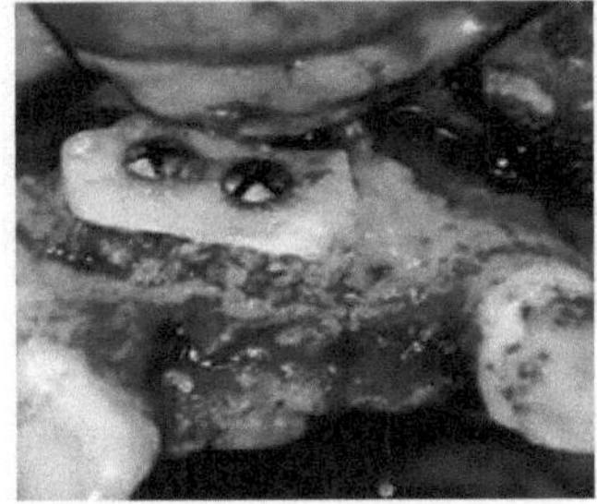

Figure 39. Filling the space created between the cortical graft and the deficient residual crest with ground autogenous cancellous bone.

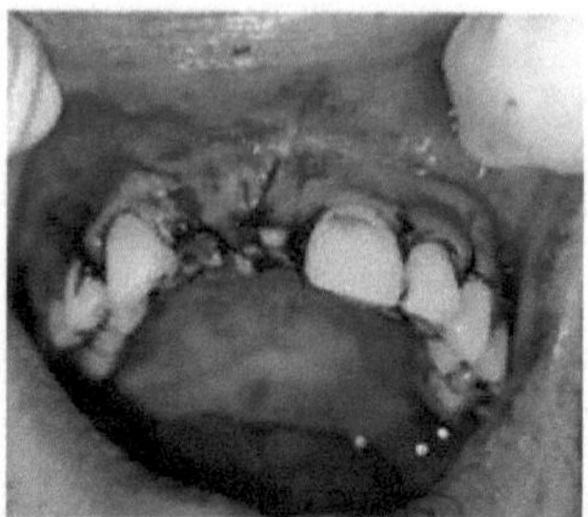

Figure 40: Repositioning of the detached flap and closure of the wound with tension-free hermetic sutures.

<♦ Healing check after 10 days:

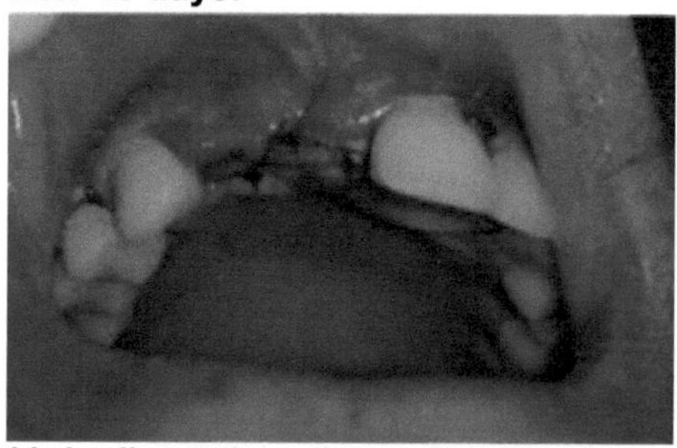

Figure 41. Favourable healing at the recipient site: closed wound with no signs of inflammation. Temporisation was achieved with a glued bridge on 21 and 13.

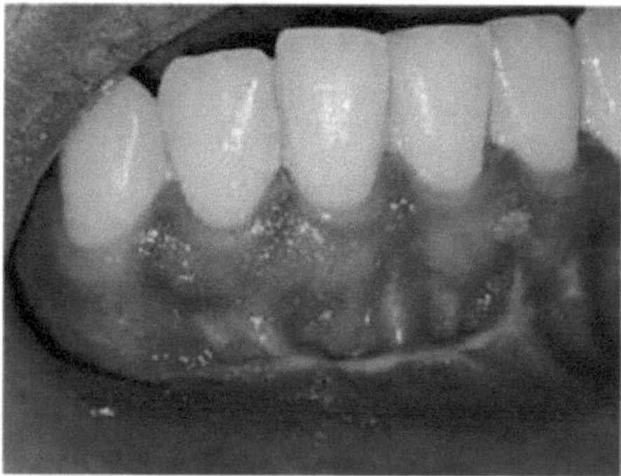

Figure 42. Postoperative appearance of the donor site at 10 days: Healing is favourable.

*** Planning and fitting of 2 implants after 4 months:**

Re-entry surgery after 4 months of healing (the time required for bone neoformation after the formwork graft):

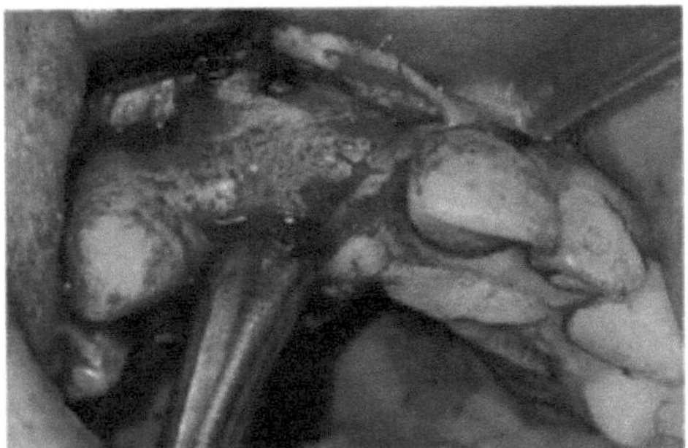

Figure 43. Significant bone volume gain after 4 months, allowing ideal positioning of the implants

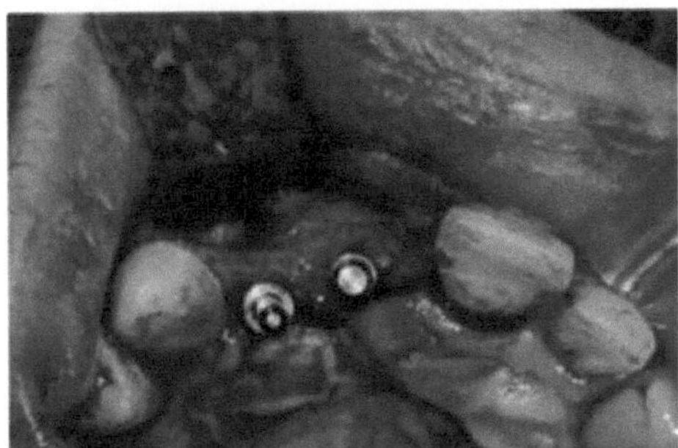

Figure 44. Placement of 2 implants at sites 11 and 12 with implant burying.

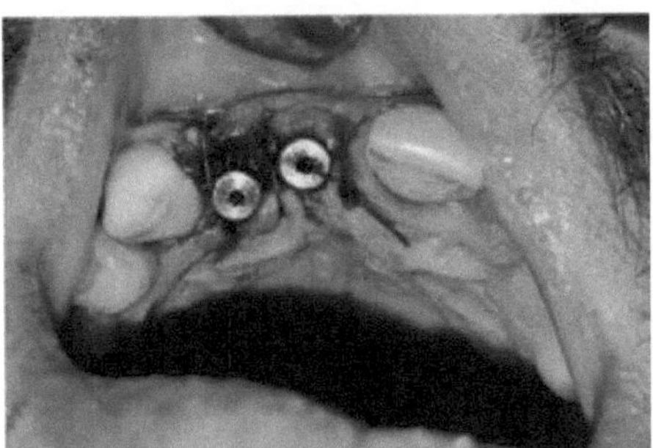

Figure 45. After 3 months, placement of 2 healing screws with an apically displaced flap

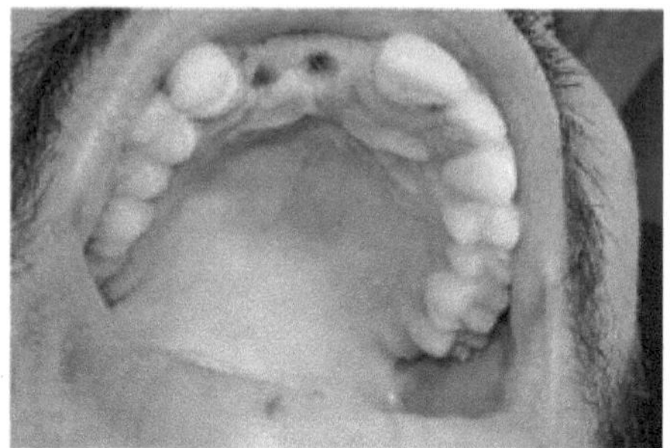

Figure 46. Removal of the healing screws: the site is well healed and the 2 implants are stable and well integrated.

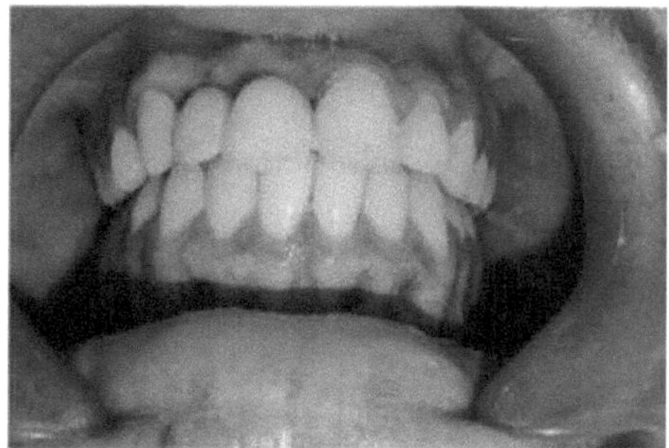

Figure 47. Manufacture of provisional prostheses in PMMA resin

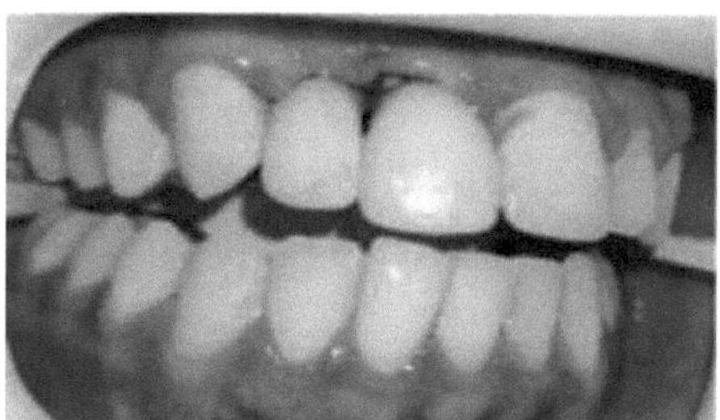

Figure 48. Clinical aspect 3 weeks after the provisional prostheses have been fitted: a graft of buried connective tissue is planned in order to recreate the dental papilla between 2 of the implant-supported prostheses, with modelling of the 2 provisional prostheses to adjust the emergence profile.

5.2. Clinical case N°2

Patient D.K, aged 60, in good general health, presented to the dental medicine department of the Farhat Hached University Hospital in Sousse for prosthetic rehabilitation of teeth 14 and 15. These 2 teeth were deemed non-conservable and had already been extracted 4 months previously.

Clinical examination :

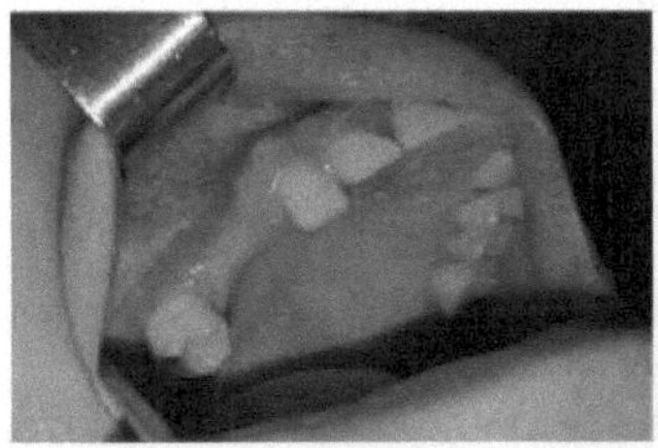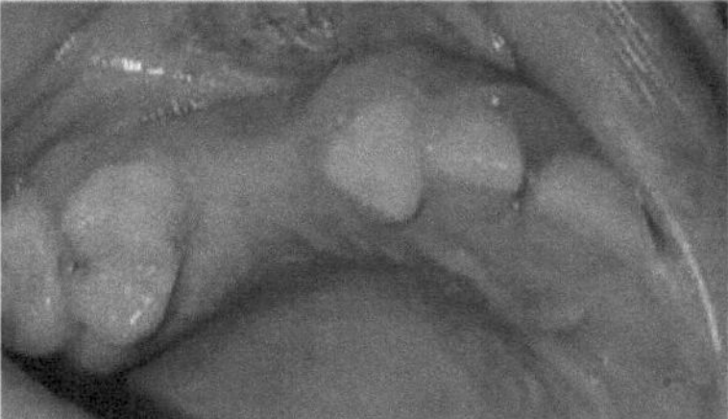

Figure 49. Endooral view of the edentulous ridge showing satisfactory hygiene with a thick periodontal biotype.

Radiological examination :

Maxillary cone beam examination showed a moderate insufficiency of transverse bone volume at the sites of 14 and 15.

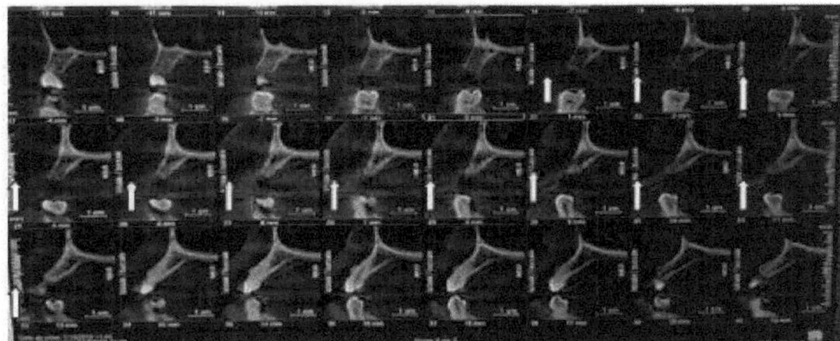

Figure 50. Oblique coronal sections through the maxillary edentulous ridge showing the insufficient horizontal bone volume at the sites of 14 and 15.

Therapeutic decision :

Implant-supported rehabilitation of 14 and 15 with per-implant crete expansion using the "bone speading" dilatation technique.

Operating protocol :

The steps in the operating protocol are illustrated in the following figures:

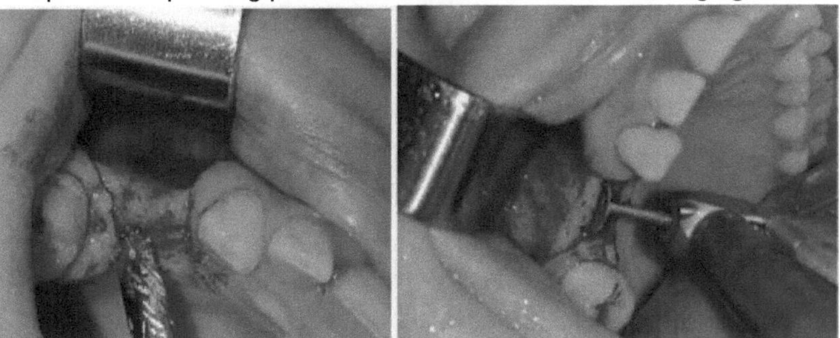

Figure 51. After anaesthesia and flap detachment, a deep crestal osteotomy was performed using a bone saw mounted on a counter-angle.

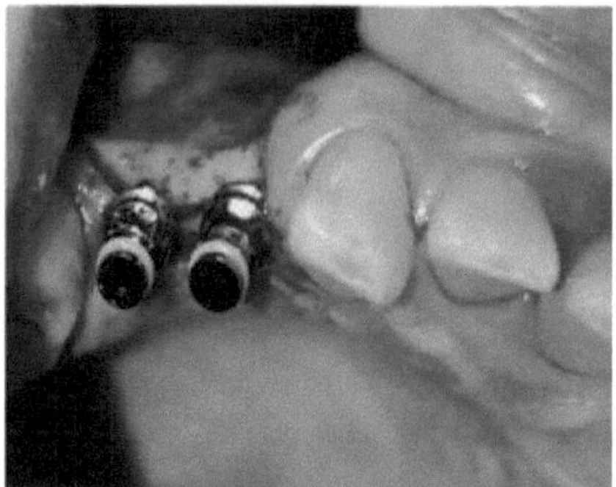

Figure 52. Successive passage of a series of spreaders in ascending order to allow the crete to expand.

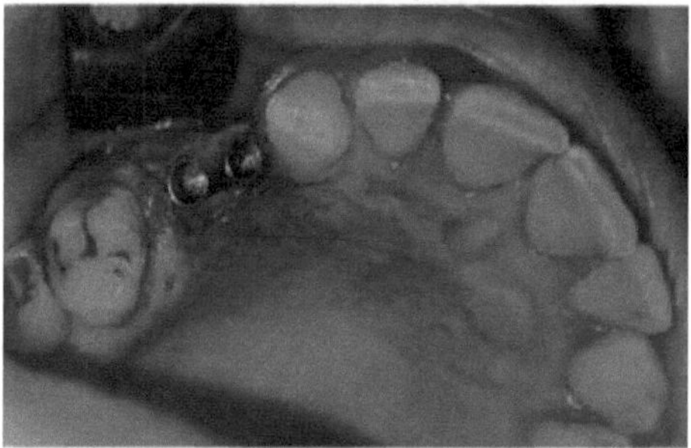

Figure 53. Placement of 2 implants with a diameter of 3.7mm at the sites of 14 and 15 after crete expansion.

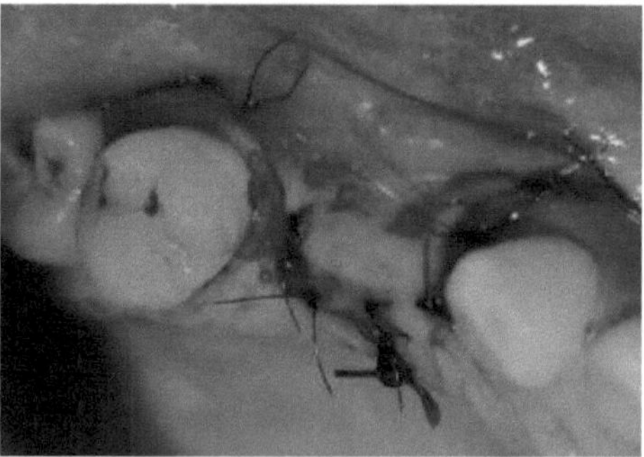

Figure 54. Closure of the wound using hermetic sutures.

Prothetic stages after 3 months:

After removal of the healing screws, the 2 implants at the sites of 14 and 15 were well osseointegrated and stable, surrounded by sufficient horizontal bone volume, which allowed us to begin the prosthetic phase:

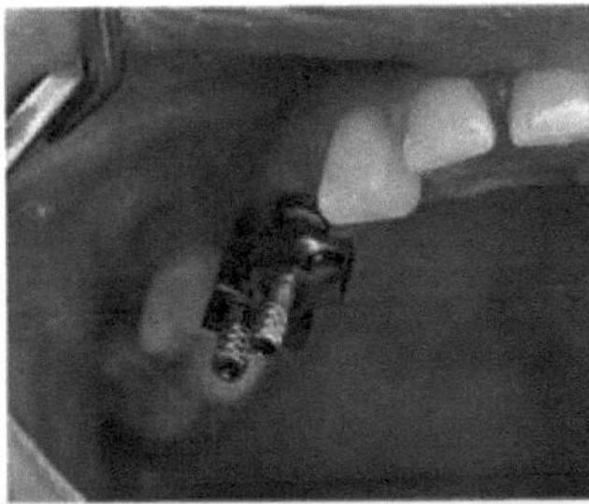

Figure 55. Positioning the 2 pick-up transfers for the working impression

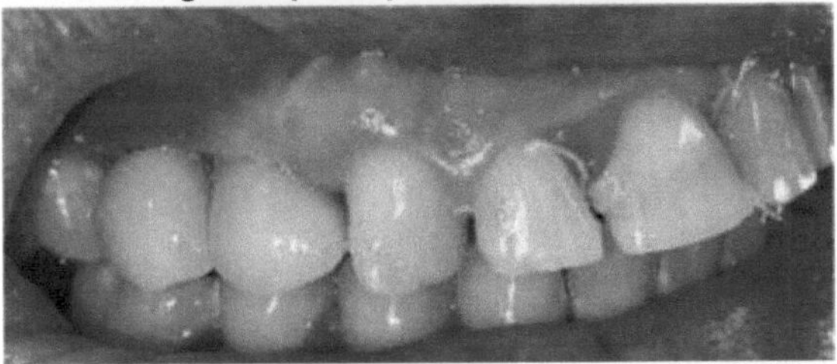

Figure 56. Aesthetically satisfactory implant-supported definitive prosthetic rehabilitation of 14 and 15.

5.3. Clinical case N°3

A 31-year-old female patient, A.D, in good general health, consulted the dental medicine department of the Farhat Hached University Hospital in Sousse for prosthetic rehabilitation of the edentulous right premolar region.

Clinical examination revealed a borderline space between 13 and 16 and a thin, knife-edge ridge with a vestibular depression. However, the height of the keratinised gingiva was sufficient.

Radiological examination of the oblique coronal sections of the maxillary cone beam passing through the edentulous region confirms the presence of a significant horizontal bone defect with 3 walls. There is a vestibular concavity over the entire height of the edentulous ridge.

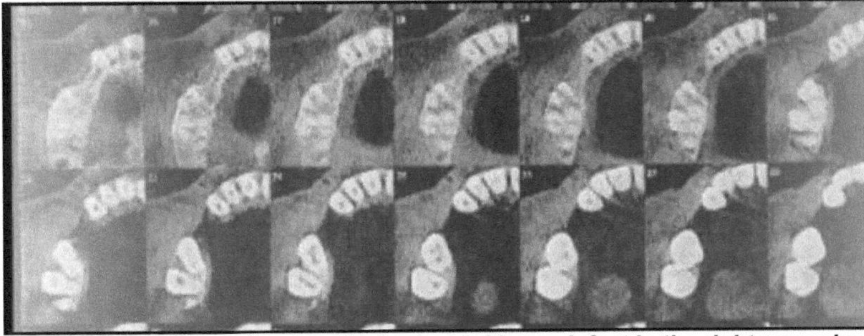

Figure 57. Axial sections showing the horizontal bone defect in the right premolar area

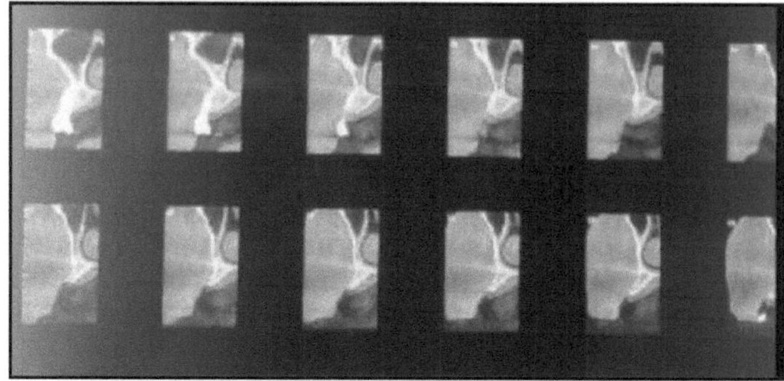

Figure 58. Oblique coronal sections showing the horizontal bone defect in the right premolar area

Therapeutic decision :

Implant-supported rehabilitation of 14 and 15 with pre-implant guided bone regeneration using a bovine cross-linked collagen membrane and filling with a mixture of xenogenic bone substitute using the "tenting screw" technique. Opening of the mesio-distal space by distalization of 16 using orthodontic treatment postoperatively is also planned in order to create space for the implant-supported prosthesis of 14 and 15.

Operating protocol :

The steps in the operating protocol are illustrated in the following figures:

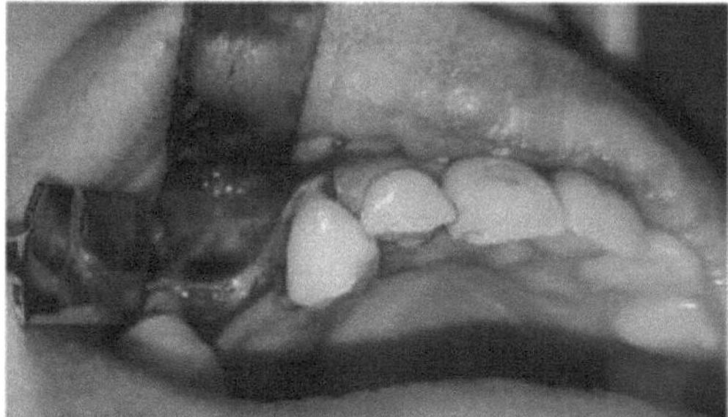

Figure 59. Anaesthesia, incision with a single offset towards the mesial surface of the canine, full-thickness flap detachment, debridement of the site to eliminate fibrous tissue and granulation tissue and provide endosteal stimulation, flap release by dissection of the periosteum.

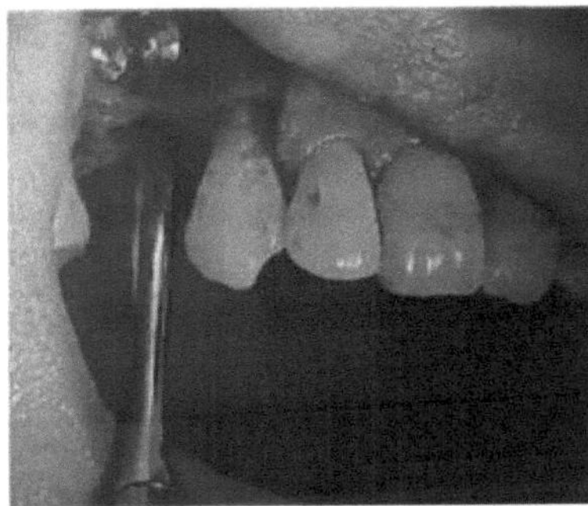

Figure 60: Drilling at the site using an adapted drill bit fixed to the handpiece and insertion of the 2 osteosynthesis screws.

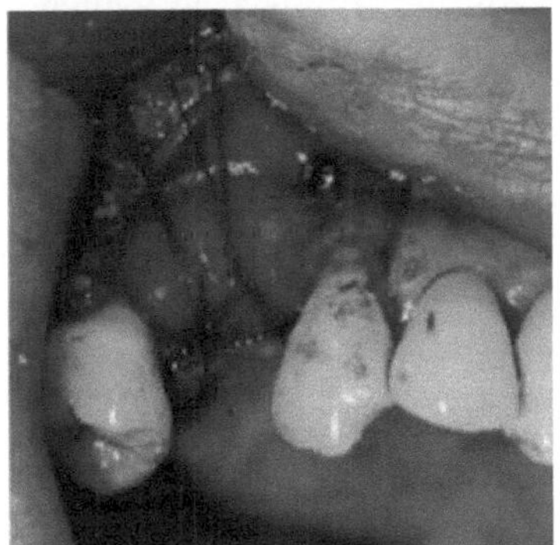

Figure 61. Filling of the space with a bone substitute (xenograft 0.5g GENOSS) + placement of the resorbable collagen membrane reticulated above with fixation using pins mounted on pneumatic pin holders + placement of periosteal sutures to optimise fixation of the membrane and ensure maintenance of the scar space.

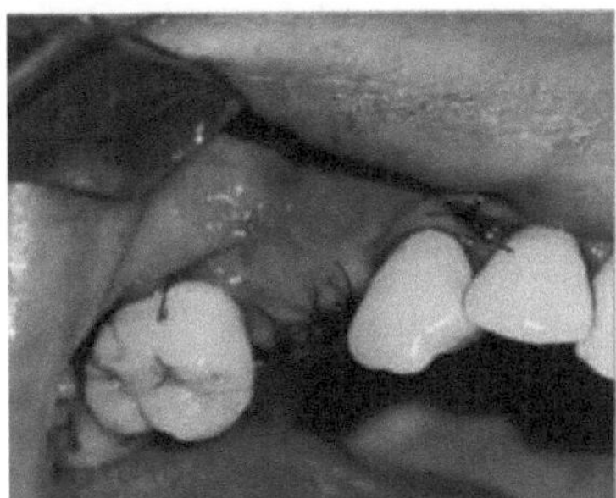

Figure 62. Repositioning the flap and suturing without tension

Antibiotic prescription based on amoxcillin (2g/d), paracetamol (3g/d), antiseptic mouthwash based on chlorexidine and perio kin spray.
Check-up after 10 days with removal of stitches:

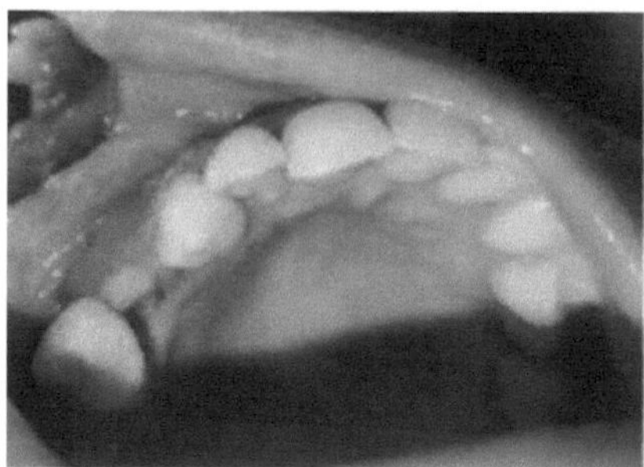

Figure 63. Clinical view showing favourable healing of the site at D10 post-operatively

Further treatment :

After 6 months, when bone neoformation is complete (confirmed by CBCT examination), surgery will be scheduled to place implants at the 14 and 15 sites.

5.4. Clinical case N°4

Patient Oussama M., aged 28, consulted our department for the replacement of a 21 that had been lost in a fall since childhood. Clinical examination revealed significant vestibular depression and deviation of the inter-incisal midline.

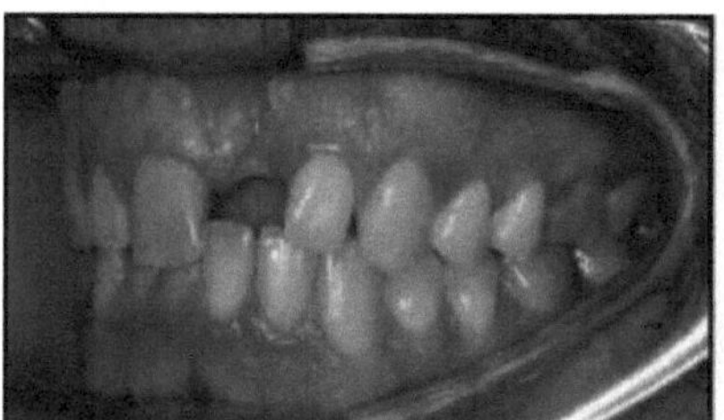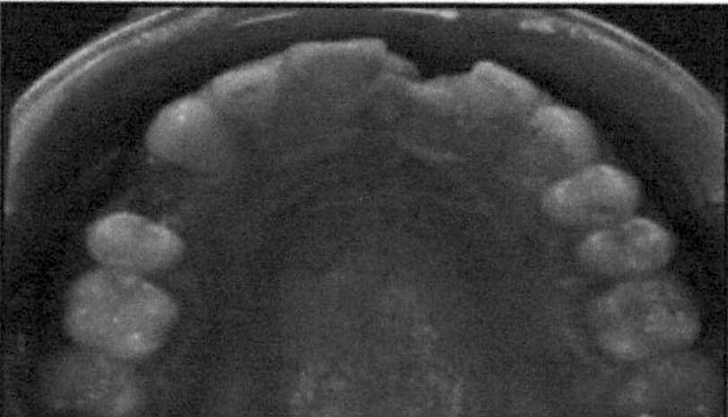

Figure 64. Front view of the edentulous arch Figure 65. Occlusal view of the edentulous arch

A pre-implant Cone Beam showed a consequent vestibular concavity, highlighting a horizontal bone defect requiring pre-implant bone grafting. Given the extent of the bone defect, an autogenous block graft at the site of the 21 using a formwork technique was adopted. The patient was also referred to the orthodontist for mid-incisal alignment.

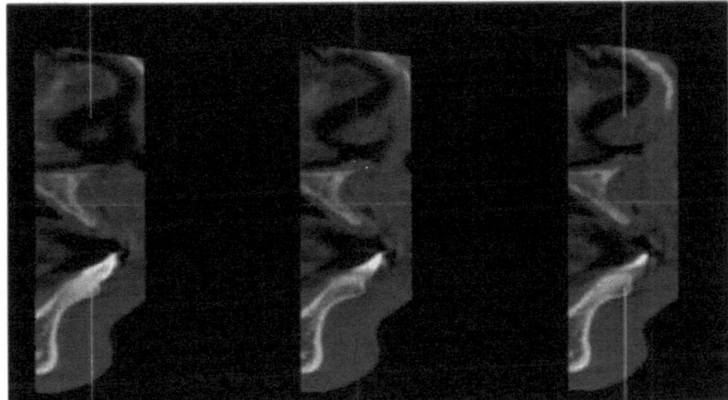

Figure 66. Cone Beam; horizontal resorption with pronounced vestibular concavity

Operating stages:

• Preparation of the recipient site: creation of a full-thickness trapezoidal flap, debridement of fibro-inflammatory tissue and dissection of the periosteum in order to passivate the flap for tension-free closure.

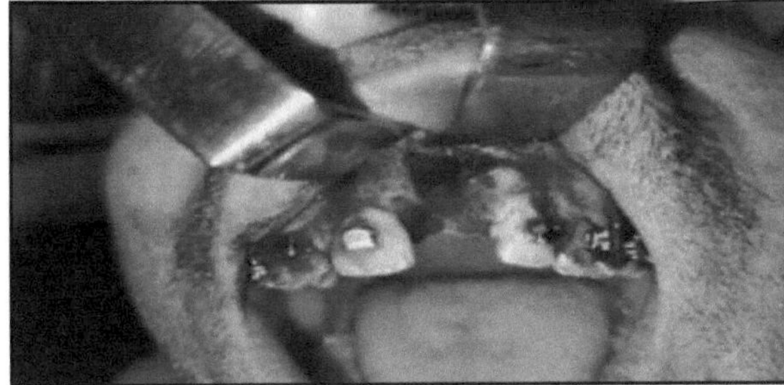

Figure 67. Detachment of the full thickness flap

• After anaesthesia, an incision was made at the base of the vestibule, 5 mm beyond the muco-gingival line running from canine to canine, and the flap was detached by freeing the muscular attachments in the chin region.

• Removal of the symphyseal autogenous bone block After the osteotomy had been traced by piezosurgery, the PRF was placed (in order to optimise the post-operative period).

• Removal of autogenous particulate bone using the bone scraper.

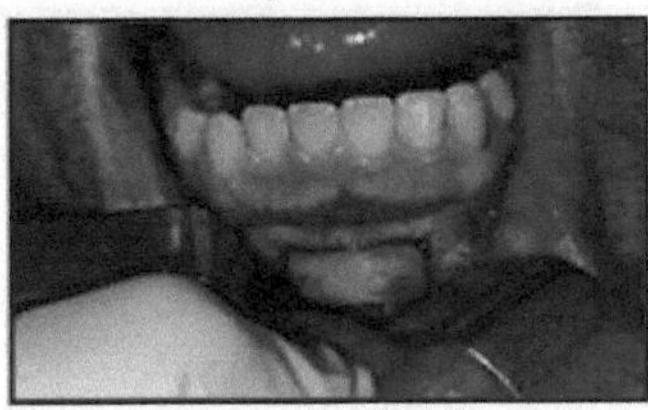 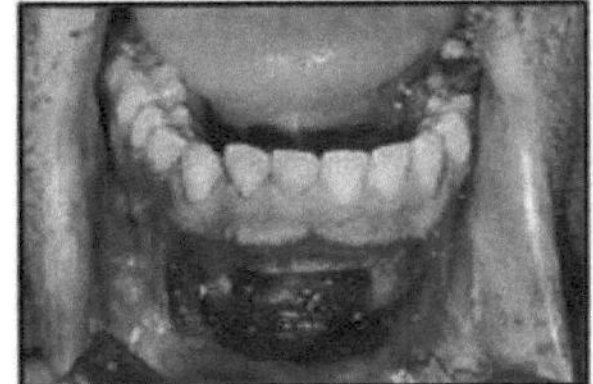

Figure 68. Tracée de l'ostéotomie par piezosurgery Figure 69. Symphyseal sampling

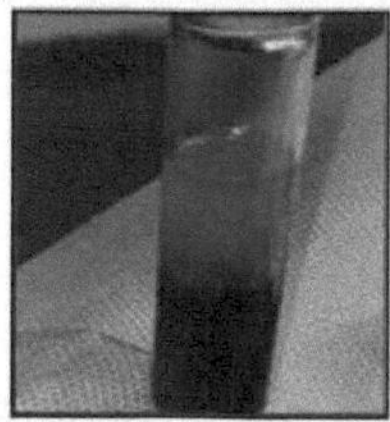 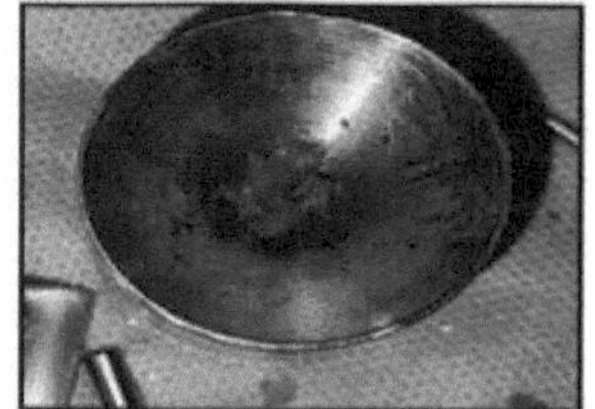

Figure 70. PRF in tube Figure 71. Particulaire bone autogenous mixedangé au sang

• Closure of the wound using separate sutures, and

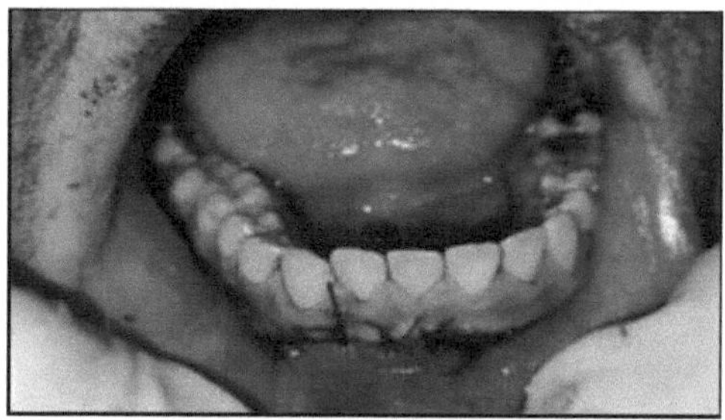

hermetic (sutures made in 2 planes: muscular and mucosal)

• Adaptation and fixation of the cortical graft using 2 osteosynthesis screws and filling of the space created between the cortical graft and the residual deficient bone using particulate autogenous cancellous bone.
• Repositioning of the detached flap and closure of the wound using hermetic sutures without tension and prescription of antibiotics based on amoxicillin (2g/d), paracetamol (3g/d), chlorexidine-based antiseptic mouthwash and Perio kin spray.

Figure 72. Hermetic sutures of the donor site

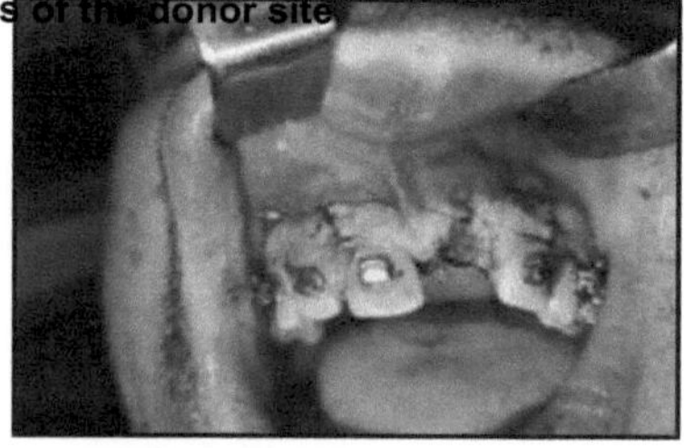

Figure 73. Fixation of the graft with osteosynthesis

Figure 74. Hermetic wound sutures without tension

- After a control CBCT, re-entry surgery is performed after 4 months of healing (the time required for bone neo-formation after the formwork graft).
- Removal of the osteosynthesis screws and insertion of the 21 mm implant with a cingular opening for the screw-retained prosthesis

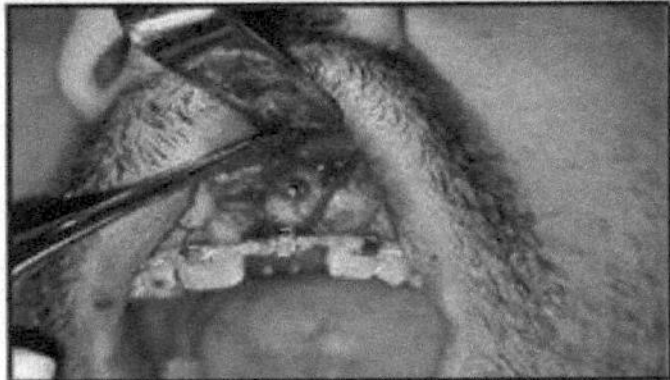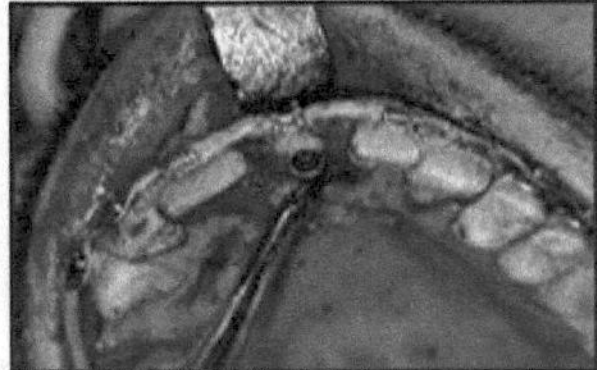

Figure 75. Removing the fixation screws Figure 76. Placing the implant

- After 2 months, the healing screw is inserted.

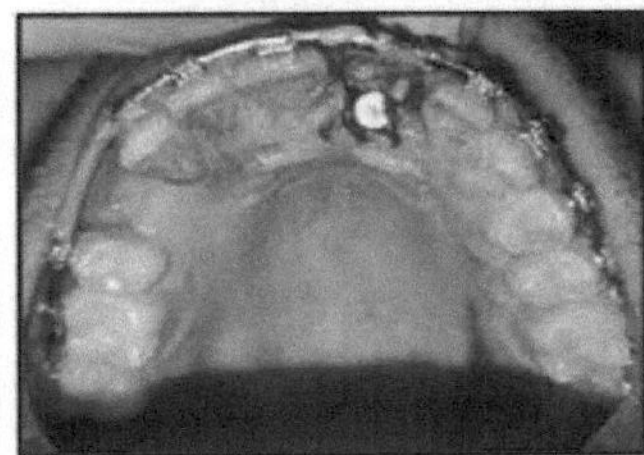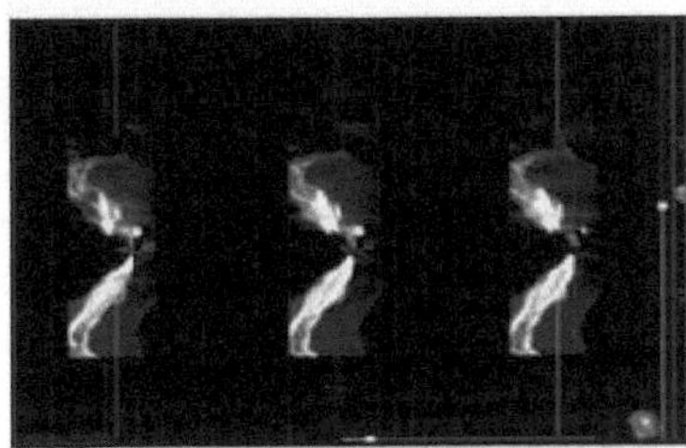

Figure 77. Cicatrisation screw in place Figure 78. CBCT check-up after 4 months

- Optimisation of peri-implant soft tissue thickness by placement of a buried connective tissue graft using a tunneling technique and fabrication of a PMMA provisional prosthesis to guide healing and improve the implant emergence profile.

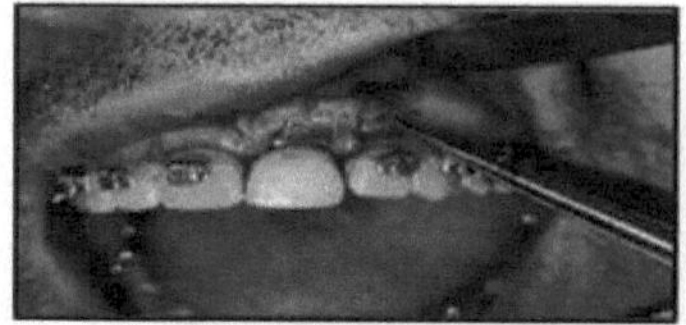
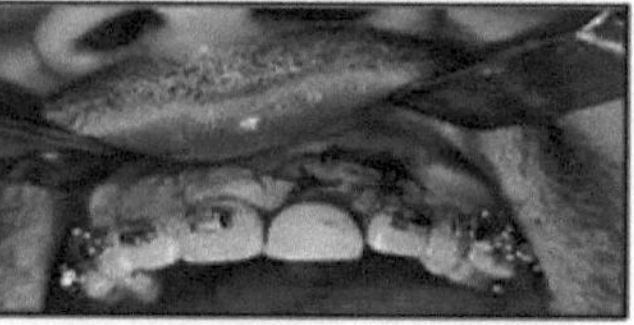

Figure 79. Connective graft buried using a tunneling technique, followed by closure of the wound and fitting of a temporary PMMA crown.

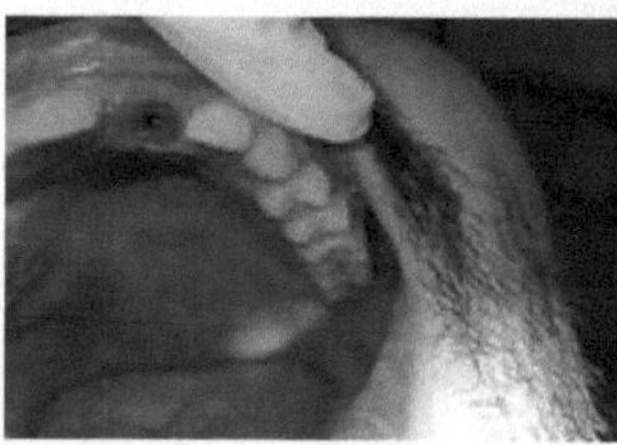
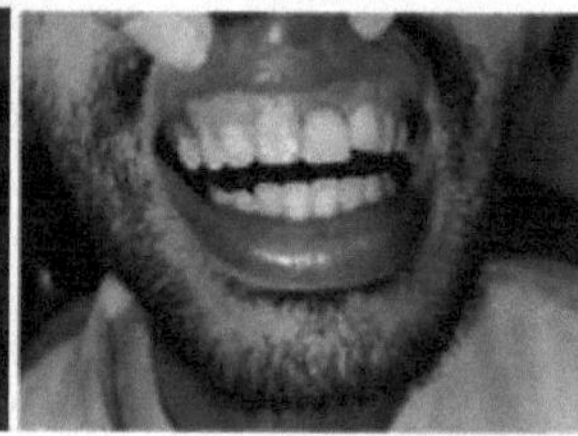

Figure 80: Optimisation of the emergence profile with the provisional prosthesis

5.5. Clinical case N°5

Patient Fathi B., aged 54, in BEG consulted for implant-supported prosthetic rehabilitation of the right maxillary sector. The pre-implant Cone Beam showed terminal bone lysis of 12 associated with vestibular bone loss. 1 month after the CBCT was performed, the 12 was spontaneously avulsed.

Therapeutic decision: early implant extraction combined with per-implant ROG.

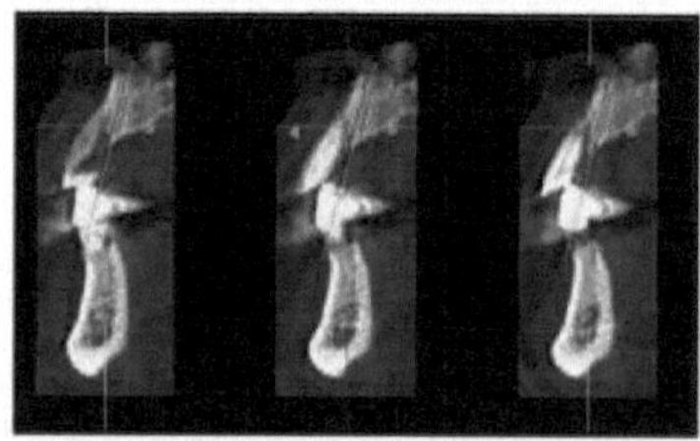
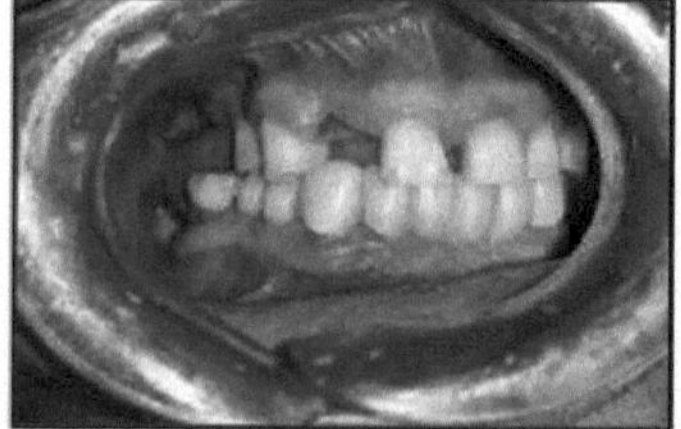

Figure 81. Cone Beam avant the avulsion of la 12 Figure 82. Front view of the edentulous tooth

Surgical protocol :

- Incision and detachment of a lambeau of full epaisseur. Plating of the implant according to the three-dimensional planification: fenestration au level with the vestibulaire turns of the implant.

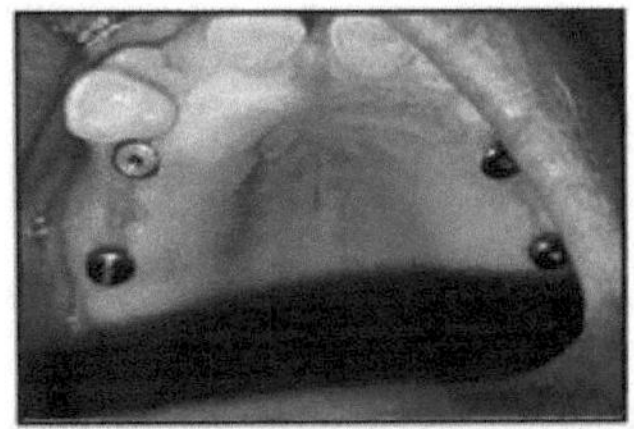 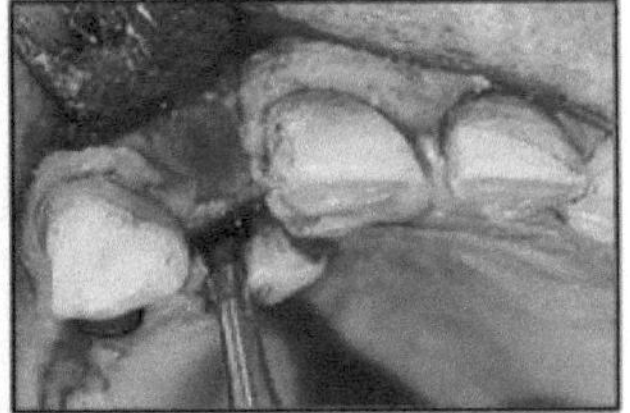

Figure 83. Occlusal view of the edentulous tooth Figure 84. Detachment of the lambeau

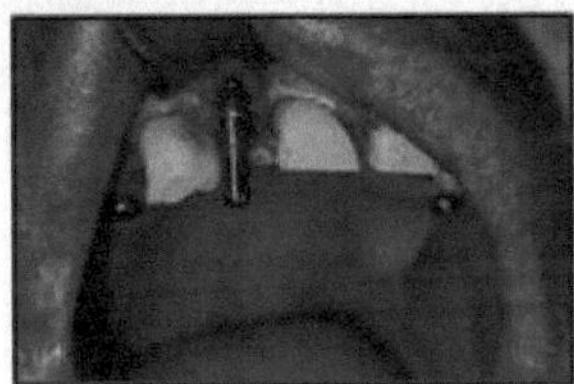 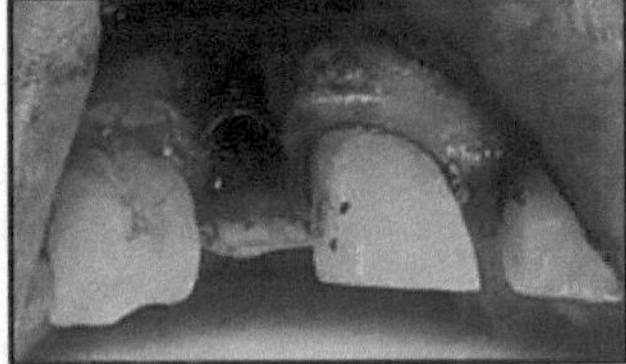

Figure 85. Placement of the implant of la 12; vestibulaire fenestration at the level of the implant

- Placement of the cover screw, dissection of the periosteum. - Filling of the horizontal defect with bovine particulaire bone (BioOss granulometry average 0.5 g) and placement of a collagene membrane fixed by periosteal sutures. - Tight closure of the site without tension.

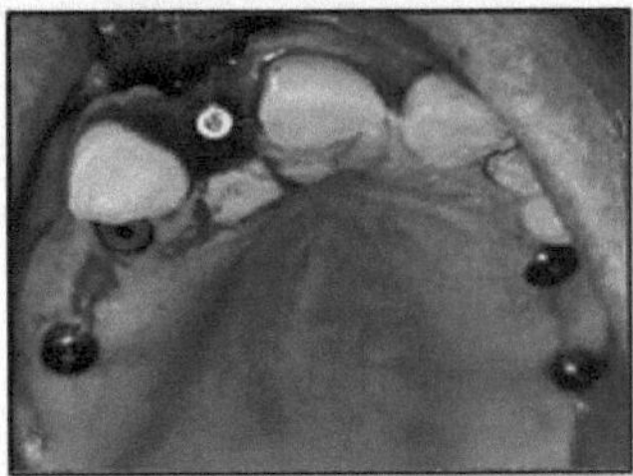 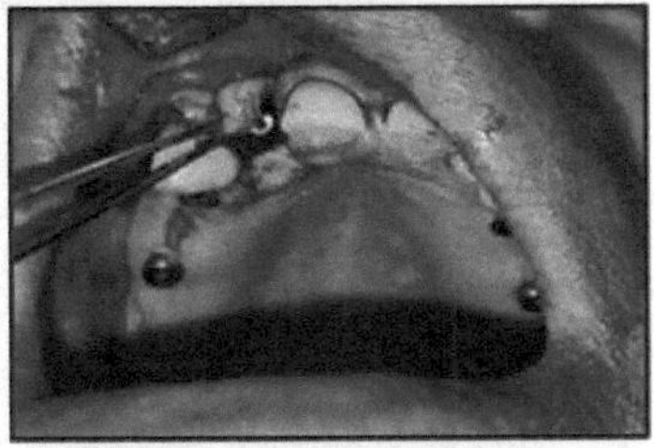

Figure 86. Cover screw in place Figure 87. Dissection of the periosteum

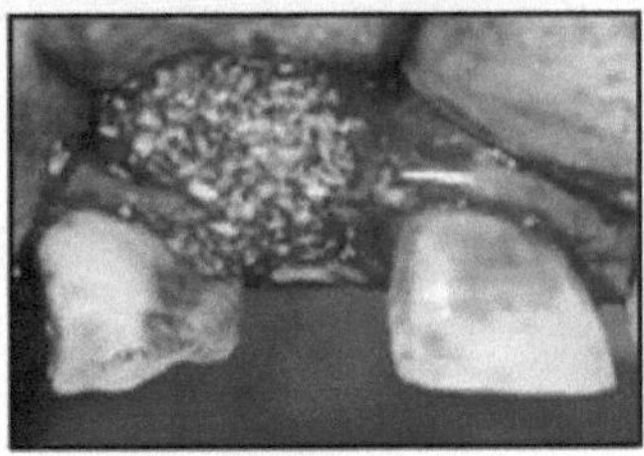 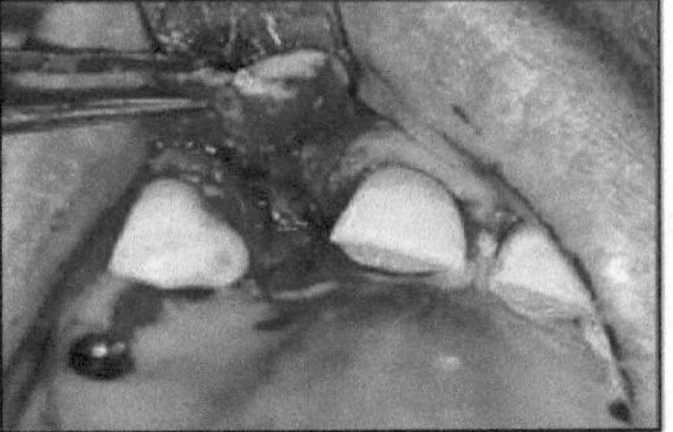

Figure 88. Filling the defect with BioOss
Figure 89. Place of the collagen membrane fixed par periosteal sutures

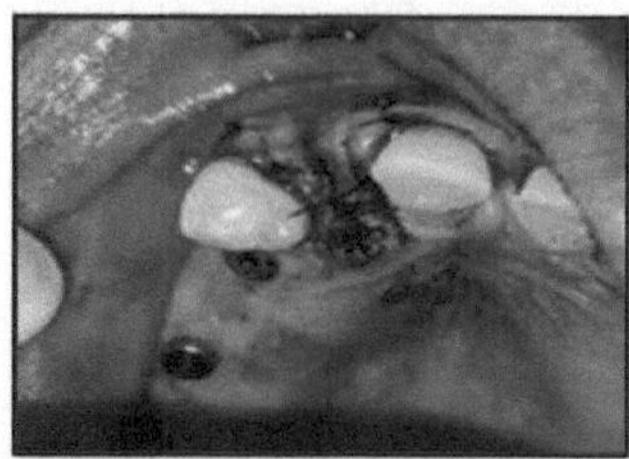

Figure 90. Hermetic sutures sans site tension - Aafter 4 months placement of la screw cicatrisation. - Digital impression taken after place of the Scan Body, choice of Ti-base and realisation of a transvissée prosthesis in multi-layer zirconia.

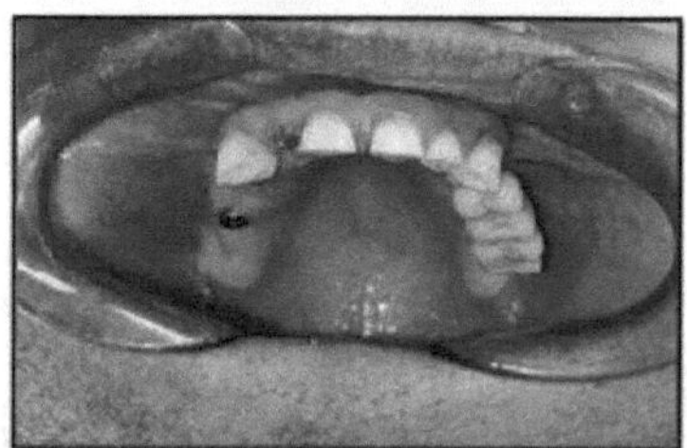

Figure 91. Fitting the healing screw

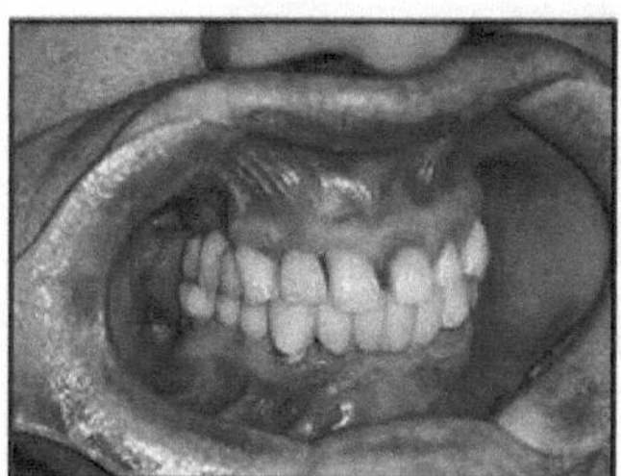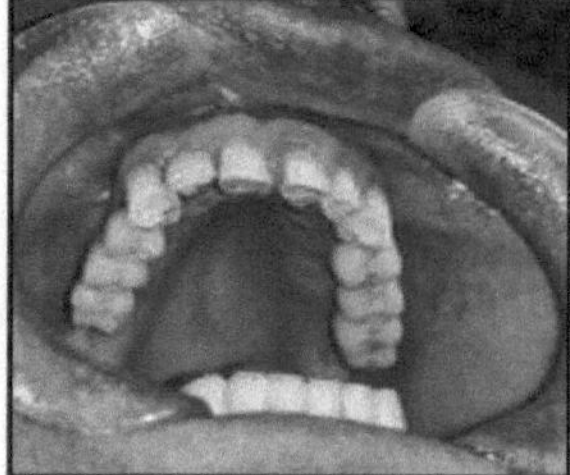

Figure 92. Screw-retained zirconia crown; a front view and an occlusal view

CONCLUSION

CONCLUSION

The management of horizontal bone defects is a major challenge in dental implantology. In this thesis, we explored a series of clinical cases and carried out an in-depth review of the existing literature on this subject. Our results highlighted the importance of taking into account the different bone filling techniques and bone regeneration materials available to effectively treat this type of defect.

Our clinical cases illustrate the successful application of various surgical and therapeutic approaches, highlighting the positive impact of these interventions on patients' quality of life. In addition, our review of the literature has highlighted recent advances in the management of horizontal bone defects, providing practitioners with more diverse and informed options for treating this type of defect.

In conclusion, whatever the cause of tooth loss, it will always be accompanied by bone resorption, resulting in an initially horizontal bone defect. This defect must first be identified during the planning stage, using the cone beam, which is the gold standard for pre-implant analysis, enabling the implant to be positioned in the optimum position for the future prosthesis.

When it comes to correcting horizontal bone defects, it is essential to compare several techniques in order to determine which is most suitable for each clinical case. One of the most commonly used techniques is guided bone regeneration (GBR), which has made significant progress in recent years. ROG consists of using non-absorbable PTFE membranes or resorbable membranes made mainly of collagen, together with autogenous, allogenic, xenogenic or alloplastic filling materials to encourage bone regeneration in the atrophied cavity by maintaining a scar space favourable to bone neoformation. These techniques offer the advantage of being less invasive than grafts, and have achieved high success rates in numerous clinical studies. Another approach

consists of using autogenous bone apposition grafts. This autogenous bone graft can ë1re harvested intra-orally or extra-orally and then it will be fixed using several formwork techniques thus offering favourable bone volume correction results. The apposition graft technique has demonstrated its effectiveness over the decades. It has been widely documented and can be used to restore significant volumes in even the thinnest of resorbed residual craters. Nevertheless, it should be noted that this technique has the highest resorption rate, as well as a higher rate of post-operative complications than other therapeutic approaches. The final technique is crestal expansion, a procedure that consists of splitting the bone crate sagittally, spreading the cortices and regaining bone volume through the centre. This technique may allow dental implants to be placed in the same surgical step, but it is only applicable to crates with a residual thickness of more than 3 mm. Currently, it is increasingly not recommended to use this technique due to the peroperative difficulties it can cause, such as the difficulty in preserving the periosteum and post-operative complications such as bone resorption. According to the literature, there are no major differences between the different techniques in terms of the results of bone augmentation. No technique is favoured over the others, each having its own advantages and disadvantages. The choice of a specific technique depends mainly on the characteristics and specificities of each clinical case and the surgeon's preference.

In conclusion, the management of horizontal bone defects remains a constantly evolving field, and this thesis has helped to enrich the current knowledge base while offering promising prospects for the future of this discipline.

REFERENCES

REFERENCES

1. **Poline JM.** Post-extraction bone resorption.
2. **Chappuis V, Araujo MG, Buser D.** Clinical relevance of dimensional bone and soft tissue alterations post-extraction in esthetic sites.
3. **Seklouli I.** Fate of the dental extraction site: Management of post-extraction bone resorption (Review of the literature).
4. **Couso-Queiruga E, Stuhr S, Tattan M, Chambrone L, Avila-Ortiz G.** Postextraction dimensional changes: A systematic review & meta-analysis.
5. **Bodic F, Hamel L, Lerouxel E, Basle MF, Chappard D.** Review Bone loss and teeth.
6. **Sharan A, Madjar D.** Maxillary sinus pneumatization following extractions: A radiographic study. 2008.
7. **Guervin L.** Management of bone defects in the maxillary anterior region in single edentulous cases.
8. **Locatelli LH.** Autogenous bone grafts for implantation.
9. **Dietrich T, Ower P, Tank M et al.** Periodontal diagnosis in the context of the 2017 classification system of periodontal diseases and conditions - implementation in clinical practice.
10. **Jepsen S, Caton JG, Albandar JM et al.** Periodontal manifestations of systemic diseases and developmental and acquired conditions: consensus report of workgroup 3 of the 2017 World Workshop on the Classification of Periodontal and Peri-Implant Diseases and Conditions.
11. **Kubota M, Yanagita M, Mori K et al.** The effects of cigarette smoke condensate and nicotine on periodontal tissue in a periodontitis model mouse.
12. **Nasseh I, Al-Rawi W.** Cone beam computed tomography.
13. **Wang SH, Hsu JT, Fuh LJ, Peng SL, Huang HL, Tsai MT.** New classification for bone type at dental implant sites: A dental computed tomography study.
14. **Fradin M.** Techniques d'augmentation transversale du volume osseux a visee implantaire. These: Chir. Dent. Marseille : Aix-Marseille Universite : 2019.
15. **3dcelo**.com [Internet]. Implant planning: implant placement [cited 2024 May 31]. Available from: https://www.3dcelo.com/blog/planification- implant-placing-implants.
16. **Margossian P, Mariani P, Laborde G.** Radiological and surgical guides in implantology.
17. **Benhamou A, Kleinfinger I.** Pre-prosthetic, pre-implant study.
18. Buser D. 30 years of guided bone regeneration.
19. **Benic GI, Hammerle CH.** Horizontal bone augmentation by means of guided bone regeneration. Periodontol 2000. 2014;66(1):13-40.
20. Global D [Internet]. Regeneration osseuse guidee [cited 2024 May 31]. Available from: https://www.globald.com/articles/regeneration-osseuse-guidee/.
21. **Tolstunov L, Hamrick JFE, Broumand V, Shilo D, Rachmiel A.** Bone augmentation techniques for horizontal and vertical alveolar ridge deficiency in oral implantology. Oral Maxillofac Surg Clin North Am. 2019;31(2).
22. **Wang HL, Boyapati L.** "PASS" principles for predictable bone regeneration. Implant Dent. 2006;15(1):8-17.
23. **Carames JM, Vieira FA, Carames GB, Pinto AC, Francisco HC, Marques DN.**

Guided bone regeneration in the edentulous atrophic maxilla using deproteinized bovine bone mineral (DBBM) combined with platelet-rich fibrin (PRF)-a prospective study. J Clin Med. 2022;11(3).

24. Maintaining space in localized ridge augmentation using guided bone regeneration with tenting screw technology.

25. Maujean E, Struillou X. Implant placement in the maxilla: A review.

26. Misch CM. Use of the mandibular ramus as a donor site for onlay bone grafting.

27. Pierrefeua A, Sauvigne T, Cresseaux P, Jeanniot PY, Breton P. Pre implantation bone graft coffering technique for posterior mandibular edentulism: Between onlay grafting and regeneration.

28. Nielsen HB, Starch-Jensen T. Lateral ridge augmentation in the posterior part of the mandible with an autogenous bone block graft harvested from the ascending mandibular ramus. A 10-year retrospective study.

29. Torres Y, Raoul G, Lauwers L, Ferr J. The use of onlay bone grafting for implant restoration in the extremely atrophic anterior maxilla.

30. Demetriades N, Park JI, Laskarides C. Alternative bone expansion technique for implant placement in atrophic edentulous maxilla and mandible. J Oral Implantol. 2011;37(4):463-71.

31. Wen S, Miaozhen W, Feng L. A case of teeth extraction and immediate implants with the application of ridge splitting technique in anterior mandibular alveolar ridge.

32. Coatoam GW, Mariotti A. The segmental ridge-split procedure. J Periodontol. 2003;74(5):757-70.

33. Nishioka RS, Souza FA. Bone spreading and standardized dilation of horizontally resorbed bone: Technical considerations.

34. Anitua E, Begona L, Orive G. Controlled ridge expansion using a two-stage split-crest technique with ultrasonic bone surgery. Implant Dent. 2012;21(3):163- 70.

35. Starch-Jensen T, Becktor JP. Maxillary alveolar ridge expansion with split-crest technique compared with lateral ridge augmentation with autogenous bone block graft: A systematic review. J Oral Maxillofac Res. 2019;10(4)

36. Fonty A. Pre-implant transverse bone expansion. These : Chir.-Dent. Nancy 2019.

37.

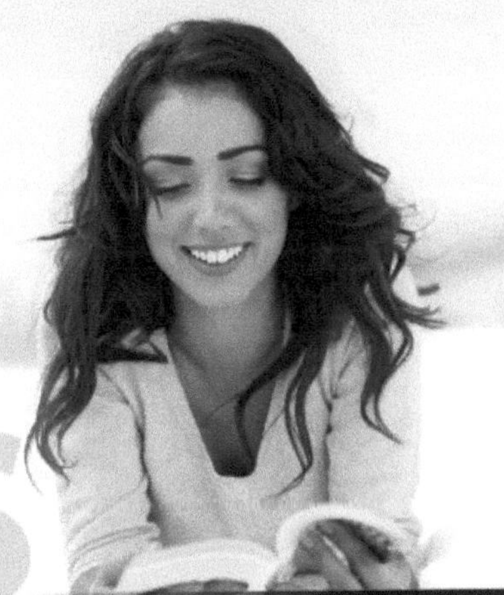

yes
I want morebooks!

Buy your books fast and straightforward online - at one of world's fastest growing online book stores! Environmentally sound due to Print-on-Demand technologies.

Buy your books online at
www.morebooks.shop

Kaufen Sie Ihre Bücher schnell und unkompliziert online – auf einer der am schnellsten wachsenden Buchhandelsplattformen weltweit! Dank Print-On-Demand umwelt- und ressourcenschonend produziert.

Bücher schneller online kaufen
www.morebooks.shop

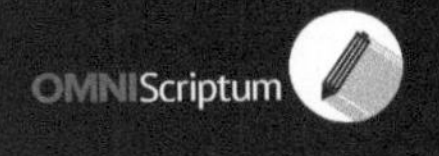

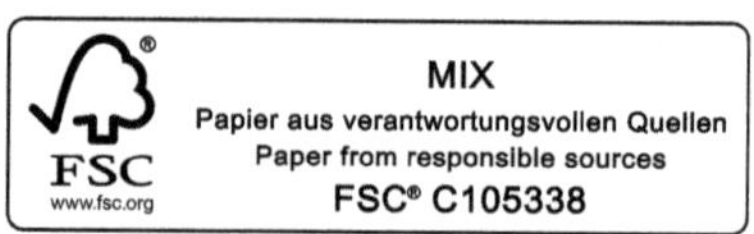

Printed by Books on Demand GmbH, Norderstedt / Germany